Dr. Dvir Levin | ON LIFE AND DEATH

ON LIFE AND DEATH

Self-published - Dr. Dvir Levin
Content editing, language editing, proofreading, typesetting, and production: Dr. Dvir Levin

English edition | 2026
ISBN for the English edition: 978-965-93397-2-3

ON LIFE AND DEATH

The Right to Choose at the End of Life
The Dying Patient Law, Euthanasia, and the Legal, Medical, and Ethical Boundaries of Choice

Dr. Dvir Levin

Expanded Edition | August 2026

Author's Note and Note on This Edition

This expanded edition was built around one aim: to deepen the discussion without repeating the same idea in different words. Each chapter is intended to add a new layer - historical, legal, medical, ethical, or comparative - rather than to explain again concepts that have already been clarified elsewhere.

The book examines Israel's Dying Patient Law and the question of euthanasia at the point where individual wishes, the sanctity of life, the physician's duty, suffering, and the technological power of modern medicine meet. It does not seek to lead the reader toward a single position. Rather, it presents the arguments, history, and legal mechanisms in a way that allows the reader to form an informed view.

The edition is organized into four parts: the global history that led to the modern debate; the Israeli history and the path to legislation; Israeli reality after enactment and the disputes over the law's boundaries; and, finally, a broad international comparison and the lessons that may be relevant to Israel.

Material from the previous expanded version was retained only where it adds a topic, case, distinction, or item of evidence that did not already appear in the new version.

The review of legislation, case law, regulations, procedures, and data for this edition was completed on August 14, 2026. Law and regulation in end-of-life care continue to evolve, and an additional currency check should be carried out close to any commercial print date. This book is an academic work and is not a substitute for medical or legal advice in an individual case.

Contents

Contents - continued

Contents - continued

Foreword

Few subjects bring medicine, nursing, law, ethics, and family life together as intensely as end-of-life care. In most areas of medicine, the purpose of treatment appears relatively clear: to prevent disease, cure it, stabilize the patient, or restore function. When disease can no longer be cured and technology can continue to sustain vital functions, the question changes. It is no longer enough to ask what can be done; we must ask what ought to be done, for whose benefit, at what cost, and on the basis of whose wishes.

Modern medicine has changed the boundaries of what is possible. Mechanical ventilation, resuscitation, dialysis, intensive care, advanced medications, artificial nutrition, and organ-support technologies save people every day who would not have survived in earlier eras. The same success has also created situations in which the dying process can be prolonged without altering the underlying disease. At that point, technology ceases to be merely a medical instrument and becomes a meeting point between clinical judgment, personal will, and legal norms.

This book is written from a multidisciplinary perspective. The medical perspective asks about diagnosis, prognosis, benefit, risk, and reversibility. The nursing perspective brings into the discussion what happens at the bedside throughout the day and night: pain that cannot be reduced to a number, breathlessness, delirium, dependence, suctioning, pressure injuries, anxiety, communication with family members, and subtle changes in function that may not be visible during a brief physician visit. The legal perspective asks who has authority to decide, what counts as a valid expression of will, what must be explained and documented, how to proceed when the patient lacks decision-making capacity, and where professional discretion ends. Only by combining these perspectives can the full reality be understood.

The nursing perspective is especially important because end of life does not occur only at the moment when a major decision is made. It unfolds over shifts, nights, brief conversations, repositioning, medication administration, repeated questions from relatives, and observation of the patient's response. A legal decision that appears clear on paper must become a clinical instruction that can be implemented consistently. If it is not translated into workable care, the gap between law and the bedside can itself become a source of suffering and risk.

Law, too, does not operate in a vacuum. Concepts such as capacity, refusal of treatment, medically futile treatment, advance directives, and prognosis acquire meaning only after the clinical situation to which they apply is understood. A lawyer dealing with medicine cannot rely on the statutory section alone; the record must be read, the reason a treatment was proposed must be understood, reversible and irreversible elements must be distinguished, and one must ask whether a decision that looks obvious in hindsight was truly obvious in real time. That is why the legal chapters retain their clinical context, and the clinical chapters retain the legal question.

In Israel, this tension takes a distinctive form in the Dying Patient Law, 5766-2005. The law does not permit active euthanasia. It seeks to regulate end-of-life treatment by balancing the sanctity of life, individual autonomy, and quality of life. It defines who is considered a dying patient, regulates advance medical directives and powers of attorney, establishes mechanisms for disputes, and distinguishes among types of treatment and actions. The Israeli arrangement is not merely technical; it expresses a social and legal view of the boundary between the duty to preserve life and the duty to respect the person living that life.

The Israeli debate is part of a wider global controversy. Different countries have chosen different answers. Some permit euthanasia under defined conditions; others permit medical assistance in dying where the individual performs the final act; still others have expanded the right to refuse treatment and the legal force of advance directives without permitting an act intended to cause death. Sometimes change came through legislation, sometimes through courts, and sometimes through the gradual development of professional rules. Serious comparison therefore cannot be reduced to a table of "permitted" and "forbidden." It must ask who is eligible, who decides, who acts, what safeguards exist, and how the system deals with error, pressure, and uncertainty.

The purpose of this book is not to persuade the reader to support or oppose euthanasia. Its purpose is to build a precise language for the debate. The distinction between withholding treatment and causing death, between palliative sedation and a dose intended to kill, between a competent refusal and a decision arising from delirium, and between the patient's wishes and those of the family is not wordplay. These distinctions can determine the difference between appropriate care and a prohibited act, and between respecting a person and harming that person.

The book moves from history to the present. It first examines how attitudes toward death and the healer's role changed; it then builds the medical and legal conceptual map; from there, it turns to Israel before the law and to the law itself. After examining implementation within the healthcare system, the book opens to international comparison, followed by the ethical discussion of the most difficult questions: autonomy, suffering, disability, depression, old age, dementia, minors, and the role of the physician. The final sections return the reader from law and policy to people—the patient, the family, and the treating team.

Throughout the book, one editorial principle is maintained: a central concept is explained fully where it belongs. When it appears again, the discussion advances from that point instead of starting over. This allows depth without turning the book into a circle of repeated arguments. History does not substitute for ethics; the legal chapter does not repeat the clinical chapter; and international comparison is not a list of countries but a tool for viewing the Israeli arrangement from the outside.

Ultimately, no statutory provision can remove the human difficulty of parting. A physician can estimate probability, a nurse can recognize distress, a lawyer can define authority, and a court can resolve a dispute. Yet the person at the center of all these processes is not a file, a diagnosis, or an abstract principle. The question accompanying this book is therefore broader than whether killing is legally permitted or prohibited: what do we owe a person when we can no longer cure them, but can still profoundly influence how they live the time that remains and how they leave life?

Part One

From the Good Death to Modern End-of-Life Law

Chapter 1

Death in the Ancient World: Suffering, Illness, and Dying

To understand the modern controversy over the end of life, we must begin with periods in which medicine had almost no ability to prolong it. Ancient people knew pain, illness, injury, old age, and dying, but their control over these processes was limited. There were no ventilators, dialysis, antibiotics, intensive care units, or modern resuscitation. The boundary between severe illness and death was therefore often shorter and less open to alteration.

Ancient societies confronted questions of suffering, the value of life, suicide, and the healer's role, but they did not face one of today's central dilemmas: a body whose functions can be sustained for a prolonged period by technology even after the possibility of cure has disappeared. The question of death is ancient; the medical management of the dying process is, to a large extent, a product of medicine's success.

In Mesopotamia, Egypt, and other ancient cultures, religious and magical beliefs existed alongside practical medical knowledge, the use of therapeutic substances, and observation of the course of disease. The ability to recognize that a condition could not be cured created an important distinction between treatment intended to change the disease and treatment intended to ease the person's suffering. "Palliative care" did not yet exist in its modern professional sense, but pain relief and accompaniment of the sick long predated modern institutions.

Ancient Greece adds another dimension. The word from which the modern term euthanasia developed was linked to the idea of a "good death," but its historical meaning is not identical to the legal meaning of euthanasia today. The Greek and Roman worlds did not hold a single unified position. Different philosophers viewed suicide, suffering, freedom, and a person's duties to self and community in different ways. Some sources treated suicide as potentially justifiable in certain circumstances; others imposed moral or social limits upon it.

That diversity matters because it warns against an overly simple historical narrative. It would be wrong to say that antiquity "permitted euthanasia" while later eras "forbade it." The concepts, circumstances, and physician-patient relationship were different. A Roman taking poison for political reasons or reasons of honor is not equivalent to a contemporary oncology patient undergoing a regulated process of capacity assessment, medical review, and legal oversight.

Even so, two intuitions already appear in antiquity and continue to compete today. One holds that life has value independent of the degree of pain or function. The other holds that no account of a person's good can ignore the suffering the person experiences and the meaning they give to their own life. Modern law attempts to translate this tension into rules, but it did not invent the tension.

The role of the healer also changed. Medical knowledge gives power: the ability to relieve, to heal, and sometimes to harm. From this emerged the understanding that professional power requires boundaries. The physician does not own the patient's life, but neither does the patient turn the physician into an instrument for every wish. Here we can already see the foundation of a dispute that runs through this book: does the physician's role, in extreme circumstances, include deliberate assistance in ending life, or does that act cross a professional boundary that should never be crossed?

The ancient world also reminds us that a "good death" has no single meaning. For one person it may mean freedom from pain; for another, remaining conscious; for a third, being at home with family; and for a fourth, using every available medical measure until the final moment. The recognition that a person's good depends in part on individual values is central to modern autonomy, but it does not mean that every request is legally binding.

The major change in later history was the shift from death experienced mainly as fate to death surrounded by many decisions: whether to resuscitate, ventilate, begin dialysis, provide artificial nutrition, or transfer a person to intensive care. Once choices exist, the question becomes who may choose. Once disagreement exists, the question becomes who decides. Here begins the transition from the history of death to the history of medical ethics.

The move from the ancient world to modern medicine is not merely a transition from limited technology to advanced technology; it is a change in the structure of responsibility. When a physician has no meaningful way to stop internal bleeding, replace kidney function, or support breathing for a prolonged period, death is largely perceived as an outcome the healer failed to prevent. Once interventions become possible, a new responsibility arises: to choose among alternatives. Choice itself becomes part of treatment. History is therefore important not because it provides an ancient answer to a modern question, but because it shows that the relationship between power and responsibility changes together with the boundaries of what can be done. The more medicine can do, the greater the need to explain why it does one thing and refrains from another.

The social setting of death changed as well. In premodern societies, death usually occurred at home in the presence of family or community. The shift to hospitals, which deepened in the modern era and especially in the twentieth century, turned death into an event managed within an institution: shifts, procedures, equipment, documentation, chains of authority, and many professionals. This change is not necessarily good or bad. It enabled better symptom relief and life-saving treatment, but it also moved some decisions away from families and made them more technical. When death occurs within a large system, responsibility becomes more complex because the outcome may reflect a sequence of actions rather than a single decision.

Antiquity also teaches about the danger of automatically assigning moral meaning to suffering. In different cultures suffering could be understood as a test, punishment, part of fate, or something that should be endured. Modern medicine cannot adopt one such view for every patient. A religious patient may see meaning in suffering that another person does not; someone else may seek the fullest possible relief even at the cost of reduced alertness. The clinical team's task is not to decide which philosophy is correct, but to determine how individual preferences can be integrated into safe and lawful care. In that way, the history of meaning connects to modern autonomy: not everyone asks medicine to provide the same kind of ending.

Historically, it is essential to distinguish an act intended to cause death from treatment intended to reduce suffering. Public language often blurs the two, and the risk of confusion is especially great when ancient sources are read through modern categories. Giving a drink intended to kill, administering an analgesic, withholding a treatment that cannot cure, and performing a religious ritual beside a dying person are not the same category. If all are given one name, we lose the ability to understand how professional boundaries developed. This distinction will serve as a tool throughout the book: whenever a treatment is associated with proximity to death, the first questions should concern its purpose, authority, and alternatives rather than assuming the meaning of the act from its outcome alone.

The history of medicine also shows that the definition of a "hopeless" illness has repeatedly changed. Infections once considered death sentences became treatable after antibiotics; kidney failure became, in some cases, a chronic condition manageable through dialysis and transplantation; cancers that once led rapidly to death can sometimes be treated for prolonged periods. Prognostic humility is therefore a historical lesson, not merely a clinical rule. The absence of a treatment in a particular era never meant that the condition lacked meaning or that the person's life lacked value. At the same time, humility does not require the continuation of every intervention when available medicine can no longer achieve its goal for the particular patient.

History also exposes the relationship between social status and death. Those with access to healers, food, safe shelter, and family support did not face the same conditions as the poor or excluded. The contemporary debate about end-of-life choice likewise cannot ignore what options were available before the choice was made. A request to stop treatment has a different meaning when high-quality palliative care, home support, and psychological assistance are available than when a person seeks to stop because no other relief is accessible. History does not solve the problem, but it prevents us from imagining autonomy outside social conditions.

The distance between ancient culture and the contemporary world also shows how words can mislead. "Good death," "dignity," "compassion," and "natural" sound universal, but their meanings vary across eras and societies. A "natural" death at home in a world without intensive care is not the same as a conscious decision to avoid intensive care in a system that offers it. Compassion expressed through touch and presence is not the same as the decision to perform an irreversible medical act. In this book, value-laden words will therefore be used only after the action and context have been specified. This is not linguistic rigidity; it protects against a moral conclusion produced by a word rather than by the facts.

Ancient attitudes toward the body sharpen another point. Older medical models did not always draw a sharp line between body, mind, and society, as some parts of modern medicine tend to do. In an age of advanced technology, the opposite risk emerges: measuring blood pressure, oxygen saturation, urine output, and heart rate while forgetting that treatment success cannot be reduced to stable numbers. At the end of life this gap becomes especially visible. A physiological parameter can be stabilized while pain, confusion, or separation from family worsens. History reminds us that it is not enough to ask whether the body responds; we must ask what the intervention does to the person's life and for what purpose it is being given.

This historical chapter also places a limit on using the past to justify present policy. The fact that a particular culture tolerated suicide does not mean it would approve a modern system of medical assistance in dying, just as an ancient objection to taking life does not mean that every modern withdrawal of treatment is wrong. State institutions, human rights, healthcare systems, and scientific knowledge have changed the problem itself. The past can show where concepts came from and why certain fears recur, but normative judgment must be made under present conditions. This methodological distinction will be especially important in the discussions of religion, philosophy, and comparative law.

By the end of the chapter, a more precise starting point emerges: end-of-life questions are not new, but the mechanism through which they are asked is new. People have always feared pain, sought control, relied on family, and searched for meaning. What is new is that physicians and health systems can sometimes substantially alter the duration of the dying process. Modern ethics is therefore not merely a philosophy of death; it is an ethics of technological power. From here we can turn to the Hippocratic tradition, which seeks to define what a holder of medical power may do even when possessing knowledge and tools that others do not.

From Death as a Fact to Death as a Managed Process

One useful way to understand the difference between the ancient world and modern medicine is to examine not values toward death but the number of decision points that have emerged around it. In the past, a severe illness could progress relatively quickly toward death without a long chain of technological decisions. Today, the same course may pass through emergency care, imaging, antibiotics, ventilation, artificial nutrition, dialysis, resuscitation, surgery, rehabilitation, and transfer to long-term care. At every station, someone must say yes, no, not yet, or let us try for a limited period.

This produced a profound institutional change. Death moved to a large extent from the home to the medical institution, and decisions around it moved from family and community toward professional teams. This does not mean that families became unimportant; in some cases, dependence on information known only to relatives actually increased. But the framework changed. End of life became not only a community event but also a documented, monitored, and regulated process in which the medical record, institutional procedures, and law carry substantial weight.

This change explains why the modern debate cannot be satisfied with the philosophical question of whether death is good or bad. It must ask who may order an intervention, what counts as treatment, how prognosis is determined, and what law applies when a person lacks capacity. These questions arose not because modern society thinks more about death, but because it can influence death in more ways.

There is also a paradox of success. The more effective medicine became at saving life, the greater the need to distinguish treatment with a meaningful prospect of benefit from intervention that prolongs a process that can no longer be changed. The distinction is not always clear in real time. A treatment that looks futile on one day may appear different after new information; a treatment that seemed reasonable early in an illness may become burdensome as disease progresses. Systems therefore need repeated reassessment rather than a single, permanent decision.

For lawyers, the historical perspective shows that law responds to technology. Rules governing transplantation, brain death, assisted reproduction, genetic information, and end of life developed when scientific capacity created possibilities the older law did not have to address. That is a reason to be cautious about reading too rigidly distinctions built around a particular technology: when devices change, the purpose of the rule must be reconsidered, not only its form.

History also prevents the opposite mistake: assuming that every dilemma is entirely new. Questions of suffering, will, duty, and responsibility existed long before intensive care. What is new is the mechanism through which they are expressed. This book therefore moves repeatedly between continuity and change: the values are old, while the tools that allow us to act upon them—or collide with them—are modern.

Chapter 2

The Hippocratic Oath, the Physician's Role, and the Prohibition on Killing

Few ancient texts have left as deep an imprint on the identity of medicine as the Hippocratic Oath. It need not be treated as a currently binding legal document to understand its importance. For centuries, it symbolized the idea that a physician is not merely a technical expert but a person who undertakes moral duties toward those who entrust to that physician their body, pain, and fear.

One of the clauses associated with the ancient form of the oath concerns refusing to give a lethal substance to someone who asks for it. Over time, this clause became a central argument against physician participation in euthanasia and assisted suicide. Historically, however, two errors should be avoided. First, not every physician in the Greek world swore this oath or practiced according to it. Second, modern categories such as "physician," "assisted suicide," and "euthanasia" are not identical to the meanings they carried in ancient settings.

The oath's importance lies not only in one clause but in the professional conception it embodies. The physician gains access to a person's body and home, knowledge of vulnerabilities, and the ability to use substances and interventions unavailable to ordinary people. From that access arose demands of loyalty, confidentiality, non-exploitation, and self-restraint. In this sense, the debate over euthanasia is also a debate over professional identity: does changing the purpose of a medical action from preserving life to ending it alter the system of trust on which medicine rests?

Opponents of medical assistance in dying often see the Hippocratic tradition as a red line. In their view, a physician may refrain from futile treatment, relieve pain, respect a patient's refusal, and accompany a person through dying, but may not become the agent whose purpose is to cause death. This position is not limited to religious belief; it also rests on an institutional conception of trust. The patient should know that the person holding drugs and needles at the bedside acts to heal or relieve, never to kill.

Supporters of regulated medical assistance in dying offer a different interpretation of the same professional responsibility. If medicine is also committed to relieving suffering and respecting informed choice, they argue, then in extreme cases an absolute refusal to assist may itself become a form of abandonment. They do not necessarily reject the Hippocratic tradition; they argue that the physician's role has changed together with medicine's capabilities and the patient's status as a rights-bearing person.

The disagreement cannot be resolved by a historical quotation. Accurate use of the Hippocratic Oath requires separating three levels: the historical source, the professional symbol, and its contemporary public use. The oath arose within a medical and social context different from that of modern medicine, yet as a symbol it expresses a deep principle—that medical power requires self-limitation. Today, lines from the oath are sometimes presented as decisive proof for or against assisted dying, even though modern law operates within a world of human rights, technology, and regulation that did not exist in antiquity. The oath should not therefore be treated as a binding legal code, but neither should its contribution to understanding professional trust and boundaries be dismissed.

The World Medical Association adds a contemporary layer to this tradition. Its 2019 declaration opposed euthanasia and physician-assisted suicide, while its end-of-life documents recognize the right of a competent patient to refuse treatment even when that refusal may shorten life. The distinction matters: respecting a decision not to receive treatment is not, within this framework, the same as performing an act intended to cause death.

This creates one of the structural axes of the book. Medicine may confront death in three different ways: attempt to postpone it, relieve suffering when death cannot be prevented, and, in some jurisdictions, deliberately assist in bringing death about. The legal question is who may decide when movement between these positions is legitimate. The deeper ethical question is whether there is a transition that medicine, by its very nature, should never make.

A central element of professional tradition is the principle of non-maleficence, but even that is more complex than the slogan "do no harm." Cancer treatment can cause pain, nausea, and temporary loss of function and still be justified because it offers a prospect of cure. Surgery deliberately wounds the body to correct another problem. Medical harm is therefore assessed in relation to purpose, expected benefit, alternatives, and the patient's wishes. At the end of life, the definition of harm becomes especially contested: is harm the shortening of life, prolongation of dying, untreated pain, forced treatment, or abandonment without adequate relief? Professional tradition does not free us from the need to decide; it requires us to explain which harm we are trying to prevent.

The distinction between healer and killer carries institutional weight. Patients allow physicians access to their bodies because they believe medical knowledge will be used for their benefit. Opponents of euthanasia fear that changing the physician's role will weaken that assumption, particularly for older people, people with disabilities, or those dependent on the system. Supporters respond that trust may instead be strengthened by knowing that medicine will not force a person to endure suffering they lawfully seek to end. Both positions are concerned with trust, but they identify different threats: one fears excessive medical power to end life; the other fears excessive medical power to compel its continuation. The dispute is therefore not between those who value trust and those who do not.

Modern medical oaths reflect changes in professional identity. They emphasize patient rights, confidentiality, dignity, equality, patient welfare, and sometimes physician welfare as well. This demonstrates that professional ethics is not frozen in time. Yet flexibility does not imply that every boundary can be moved. Professions also define themselves by actions they refuse to perform. A physician, for example, may not perform a medically unjustified procedure merely because a patient demands it. The question of assisted dying is therefore a question of professional boundary, not only criminal law: is it an extension of care for suffering, or a different role that should not be incorporated into medicine?

Jurisdictions that permit medical assistance in dying sometimes use conscientious objection as an institutional solution. A physician may not be required personally to carry out the act, although the law may impose duties of information or referral to varying degrees. These models try to recognize that physicians have consciences without allowing individual conscience to become an absolute barrier to a lawful service. The tension is especially acute in areas with few clinicians: if every professional refuses, the right may remain theoretical; if everyone must participate, medicine may be perceived as an instrument of the state contrary to the ethics of some of its members. This is a meeting point among freedom of conscience, access to care, and professional responsibility.

The Hippocratic tradition also highlights power relations. A sick person may depend on what information a physician chooses to present, the language used to describe prognosis, and the options offered by the system. Even without direct coercion, wording can shape choice. Saying "there is no point" may close a conversation; saying "we can continue treatment, but the probability of benefit is low and the burden is high" creates a better basis for decision-making. The physician's duty therefore does not end with refraining from physical force. Expertise must be used in a way that does not exploit vulnerability or informational asymmetry. When decisions are irreversible, the quality of explanation becomes part of ethics itself.

From a legal perspective, professional tradition may influence the definition of standards of conduct, but law does not simply adopt it. Courts examine legislation, professional guidance, informed consent, discretion, causation, and harm. In medical negligence, the Hippocratic Oath does not replace analysis of the professional standard. A lawyer who quotes the oath instead of analyzing the law misses the legal task, while ignoring professional ethics altogether misses the context in which law operates. Legislators who seek to alter a medical role must therefore understand the consequences for training, liability, insurance, documentation, and institutional trust.

The relief of pain shows how professional principles can conflict in a less dramatic but highly practical way. A physician may fear that opioids given to a dying patient will shorten life and therefore undertreat pain. If that fear is not clinically justified and the dose is appropriate, the result may be avoidable suffering. Commitment to life does not require undertreatment. Medicine must distinguish among the intention to relieve a symptom, proportionate use of medication, and deliberate killing. The boundary is not determined by the name of the drug alone, but by indication, dose, response, and the decision-making process. This is why palliative training is part of professional identity.

The Hippocratic discussion also raises an educational question: what should medical students be taught when law and morality remain contested? Training that presents one moral position as medical fact may obscure the distinction between science and value. Training that is excessively neutral may imply that medicine has no moral core at all. A balanced approach presents history, the positions of professional organizations, local law, and the strongest arguments on both sides, while requiring students to know how to act lawfully even when their personal views differ. Physicians do not act only as private individuals; they carry a professional identity within public institutions.

In the end, the oath's greatest contribution to end-of-life questions is not that it resolves the dispute, but that it frames the dispute as a question of power. The patient has the power to express a will; the physician has professional power; the state has the power to define what is permitted; and the family has emotional and sometimes practical power. A tradition of ethical medicine seeks limits on all of these powers. From here we turn to religious traditions, where limits on power arise not only from professional identity but also from a conception of life as a value not subject to the individual's complete ownership.

Chapter 3

Religion, Morality, and the Sanctity of Life: Judaism, Christianity, Islam, and Asian Traditions

Any serious discussion of end-of-life care in Israel and around the world must recognize that life is not understood only as a biological fact. For many communities it carries religious meaning: a gift, a trust, a duty, or a value not subject to the individual's absolute ownership. This influences attitudes toward euthanasia, but also subtler questions such as withdrawal of treatment, pain relief, and the limits of the duty to prolong dying.

In Judaism, the value of life occupies a central place. Jewish law distinguishes between the prohibition on taking life and situations in which there may be no duty to remove every natural impediment to death. Halakhic sources concerning the goses—the dying person—and the prevention of unnecessary delay of death formed part of the background to the work of the Steinberg Committee. From this emerged, in Israel, a practical distinction between a direct act that causes death and refraining from renewing a cyclic treatment or removing an obstacle that prolongs the dying process. This was not a simple transplantation of religious law into civil law, but an attempt to formulate a compromise that could also be justified in medical and legal terms.

Christianity, and particularly Catholic tradition, clearly opposes intentional killing of the sick, while distinguishing between ordinary or proportionate means and extraordinary or disproportionate treatment. A duty to protect life is not necessarily a duty to use every technology at any cost. This tradition helped develop the idea that a person may refuse an intervention that imposes a heavy burden without reasonable benefit, without treating that refusal as suicide or euthanasia.

Islam likewise treats life as a value over which the individual does not have absolute decision-making authority. At the same time, Muslim legal and medical writing addresses the distinction between causing death and not continuing futile treatment, as well as the determination of death for purposes of discontinuing artificial support and organ donation. Many Muslim-majority states do not permit assistance in dying, but limitation of treatment at the end of life may be recognized under defined conditions.

What the three monotheistic traditions share is not uniformity in detail but resistance to the idea that life is simply private property that its “owner” may dispose of at will. Yet within each tradition there are schools and interpretations that differ regarding the duty to continue treatment, the degree of suffering that may be tolerated, and the distinction between act and omission. Religious discourse therefore cannot be reduced to the single word “forbidden.”

In a democratic and multicultural state, the question is not whether law should adopt one religious position. It is how law enables citizens with different worldviews to live—and die—according to their values without one person’s choice being imposed on another. A sound arrangement should protect both the patient who wishes to continue treatment while a reasonable option remains and the patient who seeks to avoid an intervention that prolongs dying. At the same time, it should recognize that healthcare professionals have consciences and are not merely technical service providers.

Religions also remind modern debate of a point that remains relevant even in secular society: end-of-life questions concern not only freedom but meaning. One person may suffer and still regard life as an absolute value; another may see loss of independence as a severe injury to dignity. Law cannot decide which life story is “correct,” but it must determine which actions the state and medicine may take in the name of those stories.

Religious discussion at the end of life also requires distinguishing official doctrine from everyday life. A person may identify as Jewish, Muslim, or Christian while holding a personal view that differs from that of a religious authority. Others will make a decision only after consulting a rabbi, priest, imam, or another religious figure. A healthcare system that respects religion does not assume in advance what the patient wants; it allows the patient to bring faith into the conversation. Cultural sensitivity is therefore not a list of assumptions about groups, but the ability to ask who matters to the person, what values guide them, and whether they want a spiritual adviser involved.

Within Jewish tradition, the tension between the sanctity of life and avoiding unnecessary prolongation of dying received complex halakhic treatment. The prohibition on taking life remains strong, but it does not follow that every medical measure must always be given. Halakhic discussion distinguishes between potentially life-saving treatment and treatment that prolongs dying, and between a direct act and refraining from removing an obstacle to natural death. These distinctions do not map perfectly onto modern medical categories, so translating them into law required interdisciplinary work. The Steinberg Committee was an example of an attempt to translate halakhic concepts into a language physicians, lawyers, and citizens could use without turning civil legislation into a book of religious law.

Catholic tradition developed a distinction between proportionate and disproportionate means. The starting point is the value of life and opposition to intentional killing, but there is no moral obligation to accept every possible treatment when the burden is severe in relation to the expected benefit. This matters because it dismantles the stereotype that a religious position necessarily requires "doing everything." A religious person can refuse a difficult intervention while remaining faithful to the sanctity of life if the aim is not to cause death but to decline a treatment that is not obligatory. In this way, part of religious ethics shares common ground with modern palliative care.

Islamic thought likewise does not equate the prohibition on suicide and killing with an unlimited duty to continue treatment. Fiqh councils, Muslim scholars, and physicians have addressed futile treatment, determination of brain death, and withdrawal of support when expert teams conclude there is no reasonable prospect of recovery. Differences exist among schools, states, and institutions, so there is no single "Islamic position" for every case. For healthcare in Israel, the practical point is that a medical decision may carry religious meaning for a family; a medical explanation alone will not always resolve resistance. The involvement of a religious leader who understands the clinical reality can sometimes transform confrontation into understanding.

What the monotheistic traditions share is a strong objection to treating life as simple private property. This challenges an absolute formulation of "my body, my choice." Secular law also limits what one person may demand that another do to the body and regulates dangerous substances and practices. The religious contribution is therefore not limited to belief in revelation; it raises a broader political question: is autonomy ownership, or is it a limited authority, and how can society protect a person from an irreversible decision without erasing that person's will?

On the other hand, the sanctity of life can become a paternalistic instrument if it is not attentive to the particular person. A family or care team may say "life is sacred" and impose an intervention the patient consistently rejected. In a state that recognizes individual liberty, a public value does not grant others ownership of a person's body. Any view that sanctifies life must therefore confront the question of who bears the burden of treatment. It is easy to demand continued ventilation when someone else experiences the pain, dependence, and procedures. Law must balance protection of life with recognition that the patient is the person who lives the consequences of the decision.

Palliative sedation illustrates an especially interesting meeting point among religion, medicine, and ethics. Treatment that reduces consciousness in order to relieve severe suffering may create concern that it "hastens death" or deprives a person of final moments of connection and prayer. For one patient, alertness until the final moment may be a religious value; for another, relief of pain may be an expression of compassion. There is no single answer. A conversation is needed about the purpose of sedation, the intended depth, alternatives, and the person's preferences. This allows professional care without assuming that every religious person seeks the same degree of consciousness or the same response to suffering.

Religion also affects families after the patient has lost capacity. Relatives may feel they carry a moral responsibility heavier than the legal responsibility. A decision not to renew treatment may be experienced as "I caused the death," even when the disease is medically the cause of death and the decision accords with the patient's wishes. Good care therefore requires not only explaining the law but also addressing guilt. Sometimes the more accurate framing is that the family is not "choosing death" but helping the team understand what the person would have wanted. That distinction may be decisive in how relatives live with the decision after death.

At the public level, there is also the question of the conscience of religious institutions. A faith-based hospital may place limits on actions that state law permits. This creates tension between institutional identity and access to care, especially where there is no nearby alternative. Comparative law shows that jurisdictions must decide how far an institution's religious freedom can limit a service established by law. In Israel the question takes a different form because euthanasia is prohibited, but it remains relevant to treatment decisions, Sabbath observance, dietary laws, religious consultation, and support for families.

The religious discussion ends at a point that does not require theological agreement. A secular person can understand why end of life is more than a technical decision; a religious person can understand that a health system serves people with different beliefs. A proper framework should make room for faith without coercion, autonomy without ignoring relationships, and medical care that does not turn the clergy into physicians or physicians into religious authorities. From this point we turn to the technological revolution that transformed ancient questions about the value of life into everyday decisions about devices, drugs, and life-support systems.

A Complementary View: Hinduism, Buddhism, and Family Ethics in East Asia

A global discussion of religion and end of life cannot stop with the three monotheistic traditions. Hindu and Buddhist traditions contain rich thinking about suffering, consciousness, non-harm, karma, compassion, and the way a person meets death. Yet ancient concepts should not be translated directly into modern legal categories. A religious practice involving gradual withdrawal from food in a spiritual context, for example, is not automatically equivalent to a medical request for euthanasia; the context, intention, religious status, and professional involvement are different.

In Hinduism, the principle of non-harm and conceptions of cycles of life and death carry considerable weight. Different traditions may emphasize accepting death when it comes while also treating intentional injury to life as an act of profound moral significance. It would therefore be inaccurate to formulate one "Hindu position" for or against a particular act. Clinically, the practical value lies in asking how beliefs about body, soul, suffering, and rituals of parting shape the patient's preferences and the family's understanding of life-prolonging treatment.

In Buddhism, the prohibition on taking life is a significant starting point, alongside compassion and the aspiration to reduce suffering. The tension becomes especially delicate when palliative care affects consciousness: for some believers, clarity of mind at the end of life has spiritual importance; for others, effective relief of pain and breathlessness is a clear expression of compassion. The professional implication is not to assume what a "Buddhist patient" will want, but to ask what matters to that person and build a care plan that respects, as far as possible, both relief and individual values.

In East Asia, religious dimensions must be considered alongside moral traditions in which family plays a central role. Ethics influenced by Confucianism may give special importance to family harmony, filial respect, and family participation in decisions. This differs from an individualist model that describes autonomy mainly as private choice. Even here, however, it does not follow that family may replace the patient's will. A better model is relational autonomy: ask whether the person wants to decide alone, together with family, or to entrust family with a broader role.

Cultural differences also affect disclosure. Some families ask clinicians not to tell the patient the full seriousness of a diagnosis in an effort to protect the person. Medically and legally, such a request cannot simply be accepted. The more respectful approach is to ask the patient how they wish to receive information and whom they want involved. In this way, the person retains the right to choose even the form that autonomy takes.

Religion Is Not a Binary Variable in a Legal Equation

The comparative lesson is that religion is not a simple “for” or “against” variable. Each tradition contains schools, authorities, local practices, and different levels of observance. A person may identify as religious and prefer a decision inconsistent with the official position of a religious institution; a secular person may hold a strong belief in the sanctity of life. Clinical teams should never use religious identity as a substitute for conversation.

Legally, a pluralistic state must protect freedom of religion and conscience without turning one faith into binding law for everyone. The reverse is also true: the fact that a jurisdiction permits assisted dying does not require a religious person to use it and does not remove the need for mechanisms of conscientious objection and access to alternative care. The test is whether the system permits genuine choice, prevents coercion, and respects the patient as a person with a value-laden life story rather than merely a diagnosis.

Selected research sources for this chapter include Grove G, Lovell M, and Best M, “Perspectives of Major World Religions regarding Euthanasia and Assisted Suicide: A Comparative Analysis,” Journal of Religion and Health (2022) 61:4758-4782; McCormick AJ, “Buddhist Ethics and End-of-Life Care Decisions,” Journal of Social Work in End-of-Life & Palliative Care (2013) 9(2-3):209-225; and Sharma H et al., “End-of-life care: Indian perspective,” Indian Journal of Psychiatry (2013) 55(Suppl 2):S293-S298.

Chapter 4

The Revolution of Modern Medicine: Ventilation, Resuscitation, Dialysis, Intensive Care, and the Ability to Postpone Death

The bioethics of end of life was born to a large extent from technology. For most of history, when a person's heart stopped beating or breathing ceased, death followed quickly. The twentieth century created the possibility of temporarily or continuously replacing vital functions: ventilators moved air into the lungs, dialysis replaced part of kidney function, cardiopulmonary resuscitation sought to restore circulation, and pacing and medications sustained physiological systems.

Intensive care units became one of the clearest expressions of this change. They were built to save people from reversible crises, yet their very success created situations in which bodily activity could be preserved even when the prospect of recovery was very low. This gave rise to the relatively modern concept of "futile treatment," or treatment that no longer achieves its medical purpose. The question is not whether the technical intervention works—a ventilator can move oxygen—but whether it advances an outcome that has meaning for the patient.

Resuscitation illustrates the gap between public image and clinical reality. It is often imagined as an action that simply brings a person back to life, but in practice success depends on age, disease, location of the event, and baseline function. In a terminally ill patient with multi-organ failure, the mere possibility of performing CPR does not necessarily make it beneficial treatment. This is why DNR decisions—decisions not to perform resuscitation—developed. They are not abandonment of the person, but decisions about a specific intervention.

Dialysis created different dilemmas. For a stable person with renal failure, it can provide many years of life. For someone dying of another disease, it may extend days without altering the underlying process. The same treatment can therefore be life-saving in one context and burdensome and futile in another. End-of-life law must consider not only the name of an intervention but its purpose and the patient's condition.

Artificial nutrition and hydration generated profound controversies because they touch a basic intuition about care. Families may struggle to see feeding through a tube as "medical treatment" that can be stopped, because food and water are associated with basic care of a person. Medically, however, artificial nutrition requires a procedure, equipment, and an assessment of benefit and harm. The question becomes especially complex in advanced neurological disease.

Technology is not "to blame" for these dilemmas. It saves countless lives. The problem arises when capacity is treated as duty—when the fact that something can be done is assumed to mean that it must be done. Good medicine requires distinguishing what is technically possible from what is beneficial. This is the source of an ethics of proportionality: benefit, burden, probability, patient preference, and alternatives must all be assessed.

The intensive care unit itself shapes decisions. Its culture is built around rapid intervention, measurement, and correction; success is often judged by survival and discharge from the unit. That culture is essential in reversible emergencies, but it can make transition to a palliative goal difficult when interventions no longer produce recovery. A change in treatment goals therefore requires a deliberate conversation, because emotionally it may feel like failure to staff and relatives. Recognizing intensive care as a therapeutic trial with defined goals makes it possible to agree in advance on what will count as success and what will happen if the trial does not succeed.

An important development is the "time-limited trial." Instead of immediately choosing between full treatment and complete non-intervention, it may be appropriate to begin an intervention for a defined period and evaluate pre-established goals: improvement in consciousness, reduction in ventilatory support, recovery of a particular organ, or the ability to leave intensive care. To prevent a trial from becoming mere postponement, one must define what counts as improvement, a reasonable time frame, and what will happen if the goal is not achieved. Documenting the clinical question and selected measures enables teams and families to reassess treatment rather than continue it through inertia.

Medications have created further dilemmas. Antibiotics, vasopressors, cancer therapies, and biological treatments allow life to be prolonged in conditions that once caused rapid death. Yet as options expand, it becomes easier to continue with "one more line" of treatment even as the chance of benefit declines. High-quality decision-making requires distinguishing treatment that extends life meaningful to the person from treatment that mainly extends time in hospital, adverse effects, and repeated intervention.

There is no single mathematical formula; what matters is presenting probability and burden in a way the person can integrate with their values.

Technology also changes the definition of death. The ability to maintain breathing and circulation artificially required criteria for determining death based on brain function and influenced intensive care, transplantation, and law. The fact that a heart can continue to beat under support after a person has been declared dead under legal criteria creates a gap between the appearance of the body and the medical-legal status. Families may find it hard to accept that a warm body with a pulse belongs to someone who has died. This creates a special communication duty: brain-respiratory death should not be described as "almost dead" and should not be confused with coma or a prolonged disorder of consciousness.

Technology also enables forms of home care once impossible: oxygen, medication pumps, artificial nutrition, nursing equipment, and in some cases respiratory support. In this way, it can bring some dying back from the institution into the home. Yet the benefit depends on resources. Families need training, professional support, and availability in crises. If the state encourages home death without providing infrastructure, it shifts the burden from the system to relatives. Any discussion of place of death must therefore consider not only preference but the real capacity to support it.

The medical revolution has also created a question of cost, which must be handled carefully. Intensive care and advanced technologies are expensive, and public systems must allocate resources. Yet a clinical decision about the patient's benefit must not be conflated with a desire to save money in a way that hides the underlying reason. If treatment is not beneficial, that should be said in medical terms. If a decision concerns allocation policy, it should be transparent and equitable. A patient should not fear that a palliative recommendation is made only because they are expensive to the system. Trust requires a clear separation between these considerations.

From a legal perspective, periods of transition create questions of authority. An urgent decision at the beginning of an event may be made without the possibility of deeply investigating the patient's wishes, under a presumption favoring life-saving treatment. As the condition stabilizes and time allows inquiry, expectations increase that clinicians will check advance directives, family information, a proxy, and prior positions. The law appropriate to the emergency moment is not necessarily the law that guides care two weeks later.

The nursing eye adds a dimension that numbers do not always show. A ventilated patient may require repeated suctioning, repositioning, pressure-injury prevention, delirium prevention, alternative communication, and treatment of anxiety. Even when vital signs are stable, the burden can be substantial. Conversely, this does not mean ventilation is inherently inhumane: for a person with a reversible process, it may be the shortest route back to independent life. Context is indispensable.

New legal responsibility follows from this expansion of options. The greater the number of interventions, the greater the need to explain not merely that a treatment exists, but what it is intended to achieve, its probability of success, and the alternatives. Consent to mechanical ventilation should not be abstract consent to "everything possible." In non-emergency situations, it matters what is expected after ventilation, the prospect of weaning, and what options will remain if the trial fails to achieve its goal.

One principle emerges from all these technologies: technical possibility is not a moral obligation. Medicine is not required to perform every act it knows how to perform; it must choose interventions with a reasonable purpose for a particular person. This principle is not anti-technology. On the contrary, it allows technology to be used where it serves the patient rather than become an end in itself. From here, the discussion naturally turns to palliative medicine, which gives a positive account of what medicine continues to do when changing the disease is no longer the primary goal.

Chapter 5

The Birth of Palliative Medicine: From Cure at Any Cost to the Treatment of Suffering

Palliative medicine is not merely "medicine for the final moment." It is an approach aimed at improving quality of life for people and their families facing life-threatening illness through assessment and treatment of pain and other physical, psychological, social, and spiritual problems. The World Health Organization emphasizes that palliative care does not require abandoning active treatment; it can be provided alongside life-prolonging therapies and can begin early in the course of serious illness.

The modern development of the field is especially associated with the hospice movement and the recognition that a patient who cannot be cured is not a patient for whom nothing can be done. This is a profound change in professional language. Instead of saying "there is no treatment," the question becomes "what is the goal of treatment now?" When cure is no longer possible, many goals remain: easier breathing, pain control, reduction of anxiety, sleep, communication with family, preservation of alertness when that matters to the patient, and sometimes the possibility of remaining at home.

Palliative care is especially important in the euthanasia debate because the opposing sides use it differently. Opponents of assisted dying argue that society should first invest in universal access to high-quality palliative care so that a request for death is not merely a response to avoidable pain. Supporters of legalization do not necessarily dispute this; many argue that even excellent palliative care cannot relieve every kind of suffering and therefore should not be treated as a complete answer to every request.

This leads to an important distinction between "suffering" and "pain." Pain is a central medical symptom, but suffering can arise from loss of control, dependence, breathlessness, loss of speech, fear of burdening family, anxiety, or loss of meaning. Some of these elements can be treated; others are bound to identity and values. Recognizing this prevents both sides from offering overly simple solutions.

Palliative sedation is one of the more complex examples. In cases of refractory symptoms, consciousness can sometimes be reduced in order to relieve severe suffering. The purpose is relief, not the causing of death. This gave rise to discussion of the doctrine of double effect: an act may be justified when its purpose is good even if an undesirable effect is foreseen, provided that the undesirable effect is not the means by which the good end is achieved. Contemporary clinical discussion is more precise, because appropriately delivered palliative treatment is not necessarily equivalent to shortening life.

In Israel, the Dying Patient Law and Ministry of Health guidance recognize the importance of relief-oriented care. This is not an appendix to the law but part of its balance: if the state permits certain life-prolonging treatments to be withheld or not renewed, it must ensure that the patient is not abandoned. Not prolonging life should never mean not treating the person.

Palliative medicine therefore changes the question. Instead of asking only "continue or stop," it introduces a third option: continue to treat, but change the treatment goal. This is one of the most important concepts for understanding end-of-life care, and it will accompany the practical chapters without needing to be explained anew each time.

One of the major contributions of palliative care is that it breaks down the dichotomy between curative and comfort-focused treatment. A person can receive chemotherapy and pain treatment at the same time; remain on dialysis while receiving palliative support; or undergo a procedure intended to relieve obstruction even when the disease is incurable. The earlier palliative care is introduced, the less it appears as an "announcement of death" and the more it becomes part of good medicine. This also makes conversations about goals possible before a crisis, when the person has greater capacity, is less frightened, and can involve family.

Hospice is an institutional expression of the same philosophy, but hospice is not synonymous with all palliative care. Hospice services are generally intended for more advanced stages in which the emphasis has shifted substantially toward comfort and accompaniment, whereas palliative medicine can be relevant much earlier. Confusing the terms causes some patients to refuse referral because they think the care team has "given up" on them. The service must therefore be presented accurately: it is not the end of treatment but a change in its mixture and goals. Early introduction also allows patients and families to become familiar with the team before the situation becomes urgent.

Pain treatment at the end of life requires clinical knowledge, not goodwill alone. Opioids are not medications administered to hasten death; they are effective tools when matched to the type of pain, kidney and liver function, prior exposure, and adverse effects. Exaggerated fear of respiratory depression can lead to undertreatment, while uncontrolled use can cause harm. The professional boundary is maintained through indication, titration, monitoring, and documentation. When the purpose is relief and the treatment meets accepted standards, it should not be portrayed as a hidden route to euthanasia.

Alongside physical pain there is "total distress." A person may say they want to die because they fear burdening their children, have lost control of bodily functions, have no one to stay with them at night, or feel that life has lost meaning. If the team responds to such a request only with medication, the source of suffering may be missed. Palliative work therefore integrates nursing, social work, psychology, and sometimes spiritual care. It asks whether a wish that appears to be a request for death changes when modifiable causes of suffering are addressed.

Palliative care does not promise that every form of suffering can be eliminated. Refractory symptoms, profound functional loss, and situations in which even optimal care does not restore a quality of life the person regards as tolerable still exist. Palliative care should not be turned into a political claim that "if only we treated people well, nobody would ask to die." In some jurisdictions, assisted dying exists alongside developed palliative care. The real controversy is whether, after reasonable avenues of relief have been exhausted, the state should also permit an act whose purpose is death—not whether palliative care is important.

The family is part of the unit of care but not the only patient. Relatives need explanation about expected changes: reduced eating, altered breathing, sleepiness, reduced urine output, or agitation. Without preparation, every change may look like a crisis requiring an ambulance or aggressive treatment. Early guidance can help relatives remain with the person rather than panic at each sign. Bereavement support after death is a natural continuation of that accompaniment, particularly where family members carried substantial caregiving responsibility for months.

Home palliative care requires an available system. A prescription alone is not enough if nobody can obtain the medication at night, if family members do not know how to administer a dose, or if there is no point of contact for acute breathlessness. Good services plan ahead: an emergency medication kit, telephone access, team visits, and coordination with the primary-care physician. From a policy perspective, availability of these services is a precondition for a fair discussion of choice. Home cannot be presented as an option if adequate support exists only for those who can pay privately.

Palliative care also changes the definition of medical success. In oncology, success may be measured by tumor reduction; in hospice, success may mean a night without pain, a lucid conversation with a child, or the ability to remain at home. These are not "smaller" goals but different goals. This shift matters for clinicians, because physicians and nurses may experience death as a personal failure. Training that recognizes good accompaniment as a professional outcome can reduce the impulse to continue aggressive treatment merely to feel that something is being done.

This creates a direct connection to law. If the state recognizes a person's right to avoid prolongation of dying, it must ensure that the person is not forced to choose between aggressive treatment and abandonment. Palliative care fills that space. It makes it possible to say "no" to a particular intervention while simultaneously saying "yes" to active treatment of suffering. This distinction will continue throughout the book; from this point forward, palliative care can be treated as an established concept rather than redefined in every chapter.

For a lawyer interested in medical negligence, the field creates concrete questions: was pain assessed with an appropriate tool; was response to treatment documented; was referral delayed; did the family receive instructions; were medications available; and what was done when a symptom remained uncontrolled? These are questions of standard of care, not merely philosophy.

Finally, palliative care reminds us why a book about end of life must keep the person at the center. Law establishes important boundaries, but most of a person's final hours are not composed of dramatic legal decisions. They are made up of breathing, pain, dry mouth, fear, touch, quiet, and explanations to family. The quality of the end of life is built, to a large extent, from these details.

Chapter 6

From Morality to Law: The Birth of the Right to Die and the Bioethics of End-of-Life Care

As long as end-of-life decisions were understood mainly as matters between physicians and families, law remained in the background. The expansion of patients' rights during the twentieth century changed that picture. Recognition of the right to informed consent necessarily included its other side: the right to refuse. If a person with decision-making capacity may say "no" to surgery, transfusion, or cancer treatment, the question follows whether that person may also say "no" to treatment without which death will occur.

Western legal systems gradually came to accept that a person with capacity need not undergo medical treatment against his or her will, even when physicians believe the treatment is essential. This principle rests on bodily autonomy, dignity, and limits on state authority. It does not, however, automatically create a right to receive from a physician a means of death. That is the distinction between freedom to refuse an intervention and a claim that another person must perform an act.

The movement from a right to refuse toward discussion of a "right to die" developed through difficult legal cases: ventilated patients who asked that support be withdrawn, families seeking to honor the wishes of an unconscious person, and terminally ill patients requesting active assistance. Courts had to distinguish intention from outcome, acts from omissions, capacity from representation, and private rights from the public interest in protecting life.

In the United States, for example, case law recognized the right to refuse treatment and, in defined circumstances, the possibility of discontinuing life-prolonging treatment, while the federal Supreme Court did not recognize a general constitutional right to assisted suicide. This left room for individual states to decide for themselves. Europe developed different pathways: the Netherlands and Belgium legislated models permitting euthanasia; Switzerland operated through a distinctive criminal-law framework for assisted suicide; and in Germany the constitutional court intervened in the question of self-determined assistance in dying.

The expression "right to die" is itself charged and ambiguous. It may refer to a right to refuse treatment, a right to receive palliative care, a right to make advance directives, protection against unwanted intervention, or—in some legal systems—a right to obtain medical assistance in dying. The legal source may also differ: dignity, privacy, bodily autonomy, liberty, or equality. The use of the phrase therefore does not by itself establish a general right to die. In each case one must identify the act requested, the person from whom it is requested, and the remedy that the law actually provides.

Law is not merely a collection of answers. It is also a mechanism for distributing responsibility. It determines who is authorized to diagnose, who assesses capacity, what documentation is sufficient, how freedom from pressure is verified, and what happens when a physician objects on grounds of conscience. The more irreversible the act, the more central the requirement for an orderly process becomes.

This helps explain why countries that share many values nevertheless reach different arrangements. All recognize the importance of individual liberty, but they assign different weight to the risks of error, pressure, social inequality, and to the role of the physician. This book examines those differences not in order to identify a "winner," but to understand what each model is trying to protect.

Cases involving ventilation and artificial nutrition made the questions concrete. When a person is unconscious and cannot express a view, a court may need to decide whether an earlier instruction, family testimony, or an assessment of the person's interests justifies discontinuing treatment. Such cases made personal documents such as advance directives central legal tools. They also demonstrated the cost of failing to plan: families found themselves in prolonged public disputes at precisely the time when they most needed privacy and space to grieve.

Law also adds a requirement of generality. A private moral judgment can take account of every detail of one story; legislation must create conditions that can be applied to thousands of people. If a state permits assistance in dying, it must define age, capacity, illness, prognosis, the form of the request, waiting periods, the role of physicians, and oversight. If it prohibits such assistance, it must still confront hard cases in which a person asks for relief from suffering. The debate therefore moves from a tragic individual case to the design of a system that must also function in less clear situations.

Constitutional rights further complicate the picture. Dignity, liberty, life, privacy, and equality can point in different directions. One person may argue that dignity is violated when the state forces continued existence in a condition that person rejects; a person with a disability may argue that dignity is violated when society assumes that a life resembling his or hers is not worth living. No single value always prevails. The work of law is to define weight and limits and, at times, to decide that the legislature rather than the court is the proper institution to shape the arrangement.

Criminal law has a distinctive role because it places prohibitions around the causing of death. Even when society feels compassion for someone who helped a relative to die, removing or narrowing a criminal prohibition requires a mechanism capable of distinguishing voluntary assistance from exploitation, coercion, or homicide. Different jurisdictions have therefore developed narrow exceptions, defenses for physicians, or specific offenses. The way an arrangement is constructed matters: an exemption after the fact is not the same as a regulated pathway in advance, and a policy of non-prosecution is not the same as a legal right.

The role of courts also differs between countries. In Colombia and Ecuador, for example, constitutional courts played a central part in opening pathways to assistance in dying. In the Netherlands, case law, medical practice, and legislation interacted over many years. Elsewhere, legislatures led the process. These differences matter because they affect legitimacy and the pace of change: a court can protect a right in a particular case, but a health system needs operational details that a judicial ruling does not always provide.

The legal turn also created a new culture of documentation. A decision that might once have been an oral conversation between physician and family is now expressed through forms, signatures, assessments, and protocols. Bureaucracy can burden care, but it also enables review, consistency, and protection against coercion. The challenge is to find the balance: a document should record a decision, not replace it; a committee should help resolve a dispute, not turn every case into a legal proceeding. A law that cannot be implemented at the bedside is incomplete, however elegant its drafting.

Modern bioethics emerged from this transformation. A physician, lawyer, philosopher, nurse, social worker, and religious adviser may all sit around the same question. The multiplicity of voices itself reflects the recognition that no single profession holds all the knowledge required. The physician understands what is likely to happen to the body; the lawyer knows what the law permits; the philosopher clarifies values; and the patient knows what matters in his or her own life. The strongest decisions are created when these roles remain distinct and all of these voices are heard, rather than when one discipline takes control of the others.

From Paternalism to Shared Decision-Making

The traditional medical model often assumed that the physician, as the holder of knowledge, knew what was best for the patient and could therefore decide on the patient's behalf. The modern model gave increasing weight to informed consent and autonomy. Yet the move away from paternalism should not produce the opposite extreme, in which the physician simply presents a menu and tells the patient to choose alone. Shared decision-making seeks to combine medical expertise with the individual's expertise in his or her own life and values.

At the end of life this combination is especially important. A physician may explain that a treatment offers a ten percent chance of extending life by several months, at the price of hospitalizations and adverse effects. The physician cannot know whether that ten percent chance is worth the price to this particular patient. One person may wish to try at almost any cost in order to reach a family event; another may prefer a shorter period at home. The clinical data do not change, but the decision can change because the values differ.

Shared decision-making also requires a professional recommendation. Many patients do not want to bear alone the feeling that they have "chosen death." A physician can say, "Given what you have told me matters to you and the likelihood of benefit from this treatment, I recommend that we not begin it." Such a recommendation is not paternalistic if it is grounded in the medical evidence and the patient's values and still leaves room for disagreement.

Legally, this model is consistent with the idea that consent is a process rather than a signature. Material information must be provided, understanding should be assessed, and questions must be possible. When several reasonable alternatives exist, they should be presented without manipulation. Framing itself can affect a decision: saying "there is a ten percent chance of success" is psychologically different from saying "in ninety percent of cases it does not succeed," even though the numbers are identical.

At the end of life there is also the problem of overload. A patient may be in pain, exhausted, or overwhelmed. There is no requirement to deliver a complete medical lecture in one meeting. Information can be divided into stages, clinicians can ask how much the person wants to know, and family members can be included with the patient's permission. Adapting communication is not a reduction of autonomy; it is one of the conditions for making autonomy real.

The historical movement toward partnership explains why modern law gives substantial weight to the patient's wishes while still preserving a place for professional judgment. It also provides the basis for a distinction that will recur throughout the book: a right to refuse treatment is not the same as a right to demand any intervention. Partnership operates within the boundaries of professional practice and law.

From the legal history of refusal and intervention we can move to the broader framework that emerged during the twentieth century: bioethics. It gave end-of-life controversies an institutional language of rights, duties, capacity, benefit, and professional limits.

From Natural Death to Regulated Death: The Birth of End-of-Life Bioethics

The bioethics of end-of-life care developed as part of a broader movement limiting medical paternalism. After the Second World War, the development of rules for research involving human beings, patients' rights, and informed consent moved the patient from the position of passive recipient to participant in decision-making. At the end of life this shift was especially dramatic, because the decision concerns not merely a side effect or a risk but whether to continue an intervention capable of postponing death. Autonomy therefore became one of the central principles, but it was never the only principle.

The four principles commonly associated with medical bioethics—autonomy, beneficence, non-maleficence, and justice—do not provide a formula that automatically generates an answer. At the end of life they can conflict openly. Respecting a person's request to avoid treatment may serve autonomy and reduce harm, while a physician may believe that treatment still offers benefit. Justice may require equal access to services while also raising questions about allocation of resources. The strength of the principles is that they force us to identify what is at stake; their limitation is that they do not determine in advance the weight that each value should carry in a particular case.

Hospital ethics committees were created in part to provide a framework for disagreements that cannot be resolved by clinical judgment alone. They differ from courts: their purpose is generally not to determine fault but to help clarify values, authority, and possible courses of action. Their advantages include proximity to the case and relative speed; their risks include dependence on the institution in which they operate. A strong committee is multidisciplinary, hears the patient or representative, records the reasoning behind its advice, and understands the limits of its authority.

One of bioethics' important contributions is the concept of "goals of care." Instead of beginning with the question whether a particular procedure should be performed, the discussion begins with the outcome that care is intended to achieve. If the goal is to return home and communicate, a particular treatment may fit that goal; if it can only prolong a deeply sedated hospital stay without a meaningful possibility of recovery, its significance is different. A goals-of-care conversation reduces the risk that a decision will be reduced to a technical choice among devices. It also allows a person to express values without knowing the names of every medication and procedure in advance.

Modern bioethics also has to live with uncertainty. Physicians cannot always know whether a patient will recover, how long the person will live, or how a future functional state will be experienced. Healthy people do not necessarily know how they would feel if they became dependent on others. Research on adaptation to disability has shown that people may predict a future state pessimistically and later find quality and meaning in that same state. A sound decision therefore does not require certainty that medicine cannot provide. It requires disclosure of the range of possibilities, the degree of confidence in the prognosis, and planned points for reassessment.

The relationship between autonomy and relationships has also been criticized and refined. A model of an entirely independent individual making decisions alone does not fit every culture or every family. Some people want their children to decide together with them; others do not want full prognostic information and prefer it to be shared with a relative. Respect for autonomy can include respect for a person's decision to involve others. But "culture" must never become an excuse for silencing the person. The patient should be asked how information and decisions are to be managed.

The concept of the "patient's best interests" has changed as well. In the past it was defined largely by the physician; today it combines professional knowledge with the individual's own values. A physician can estimate whether treatment is likely to prolong life, but cannot alone determine whether additional months in a state of total dependence are a desirable outcome for a particular person. At the same time, a personal preference cannot turn ineffective treatment into effective treatment. Bioethics therefore describes a partnership: professionals define what is clinically possible and reasonable, and the patient chooses among those possibilities according to his or her values.

End-of-life bioethics has also expanded from the treatment room into public policy. The availability of hospice, access to advance directives, staff training, and inequality are not problems of a single case. A society can proclaim autonomy while requiring complicated forms, providing information in only one language, or concentrating services in major centers. The success of legislation should therefore be measured not only by whether individual decisions are legally correct, but also by who can actually use the mechanisms and who remains outside them.

End-of-life care also shows why ethics cannot remain solely in the hands of experts. Ultimately, citizens are the people who live through these decisions. Professional language that the public cannot understand reduces the ability to plan in advance. A book, a community discussion, or an explanation by a family physician can be part of public ethics: they allow people to think about preferences before an emergency admission. In this sense, knowledge becomes a protective mechanism, not merely academic material.

Having established the historical, professional, religious, technological, palliative, and bioethical foundations, the discussion can now move forward without repeatedly rebuilding them. The next stage will focus on concepts. The question will no longer be where the controversy came from, but what exactly we mean when we speak of a terminal patient, brain death, life-prolonging treatment, sedation, euthanasia, and assistance in dying. Linguistic precision is the condition for ensuring that the remainder of the book does not proceed through emotionally charged words that conceal different acts.

Chapter 7

From Proposals for Euthanasia to Eugenics and Nazism

The nineteenth century changed the debate because medicine acquired more effective tools for controlling pain and consciousness. The development of anesthetic agents and the medical use of opiates made the possibility of causing a quiet and rapid death more practically conceivable rather than merely philosophical. Once a physician can dramatically reduce pain, the question naturally arises as to where the boundary lies between pain treatment and the use of medical knowledge to shorten life.

In 1870, the English teacher and thinker Samuel Williams proposed that, in cases of incurable illness and severe suffering, anesthetic substances might be used at the patient's request to bring about death quickly and without pain. The proposal is regarded as a landmark because it already contains features recognizable in the modern debate: an incurable condition, suffering, a request by the patient, and the use of a medical means to cause death.

From this point onward, the question increasingly became political and legal. At the beginning of the twentieth century, various initiatives were introduced in the United States and Britain to permit euthanasia under defined conditions. They did not at that time establish a stable legal regime, but the very fact that the issue was debated in legislatures and public organizations marked a change: what had once been primarily a philosophical or religious question became a proposal to regulate medical authority through law.

At the same time, a very different and dangerous process was unfolding. Eugenic ideas, which gained influence in parts of the Western world in the late nineteenth and early twentieth centuries, shifted the focus away from an individual who asks to die and toward a society that judges the "quality" of other people's lives. Once the question of personal suffering was replaced by the question of which human beings were desirable to society, the moral starting point changed entirely. The issue was no longer the patient's liberty, but the power of institutions.

The murderous extreme of this process appeared in Nazi Germany. Under Aktion T4, which began in 1939, the Nazi regime systematically killed people with disabilities and patients confined in institutions. The regime used the term "euthanasia" as linguistic camouflage, but these killings were not voluntary euthanasia. Many victims did not ask to die, did not consent, and were not selected because of suffering they themselves described as intolerable. They were murdered because the state classified their lives as a burden or as lives without value.

This chapter in Nazi history left an especially deep scar on medical ethics. It demonstrated how the language of medicine and compassion can be distorted when the state or an institution claims authority to decide whose life is worth living. Later debates over legalizing assistance in dying therefore required supporters of regulation to emphasize free will, decision-making capacity, explicit consent, external review, and safeguards for vulnerable populations. Opponents, in turn, saw the same history as a warning against any expansion of medical authority to cause death.

Historically, the distinction between these phenomena is essential. Aktion T4 was not a precedent for voluntary euthanasia; it was institutionalized murder under medical cover. It remains relevant to the debate, however, because it sharpened the need for limits, oversight, and equal recognition of human worth. From that point onward, end-of-life policy could no longer be discussed solely in the language of compassion toward the patient. It also had to address power relations and the state's duty to protect those whose voices are weak.

Chapter 8

Death, Consciousness, and Legal Identity: Brain Death, Cardiac Death, Coma, Disorders of Consciousness, and Neurodegenerative Disease

Why the Medical Distinction Comes Before the Moral Debate

End-of-life discussions often use the same language for medical states that are fundamentally different. A person who has been declared dead, a person in a coma, a person in a state of wakefulness without behavioral evidence of awareness, a person in a minimally conscious state, and a person living with advanced neurodegenerative disease are not points along a single continuum ranging from "more dead" to "more alive." These are distinct medical categories with different implications for prognosis, communication, capacity, rehabilitation, and applicable law. Before asking whether treatment should be continued, withheld, or guided by an earlier instruction, we must first know what state the person is in and what can be established with confidence.

Precision is especially important because technology can preserve a heartbeat, body warmth, and visible chest movement after brain-respiratory death has been determined. In the opposite direction, profound motor disability can make a living, alert, and fully capable person appear unable to take part in a decision. Outward appearance is not diagnosis. Lack of speech does not mean lack of thought, open eyes do not necessarily prove awareness, and mechanical ventilation does not by itself establish whether a person is alive or dead. This is one of the areas in which precise medical language protects rights.

Cardiac Death and Brain-Respiratory Death: Two Routes to Determining Death

The historically familiar route to determining death is the irreversible cessation of circulation and breathing. When the heart stops and there is no blood flow capable of sustaining the organs, the body rapidly loses the capacity to maintain life. Modern intensive care created an additional route: death may also be determined while the heart continues to beat with mechanical ventilation and other support, if all functions of the brain, including the functions of the brainstem, have been completely and irreversibly lost.

In Israel, the matter is regulated by the Brain-Respiratory Death Law, 5768-2008, together with dedicated procedures. The Ministry of Health makes clear that determination of brain-respiratory death is not an estimate of the chances of recovery; it is a determination that the person is dead. It is carried out in a hospital through a structured process by specialist physicians who have undergone specific training, with separation from the direct treating team and from those involved in transplantation. The determination includes clinical examination and an instrumental test intended to demonstrate the absence of the functions required by law. This structure reflects an important principle: the more final the determination, the more the process must be protected from a single impression or from another institutional interest.

The separation between the determination of death and transplantation is also essential to public trust. Organ donation may become possible after brain-respiratory death has been determined, but the possibility of donation must never be the reason for that determination. The institutional logic runs in the opposite direction: death is first determined according to independent medical and legal criteria; only afterward, where relevant and where the required consent exists, is donation considered. When this sequence is explained to the family, there is less risk that the continuing heartbeat and warmth will be understood as evidence that the team wishes to "stop treatment in a living person."

Brain Death Is Not Coma and Is Not a Minimally Conscious State

Coma is a state of absent wakefulness and absent awareness, but a person in a coma is alive. It may result from brain injury, poisoning, metabolic disturbance, stroke, infection, or other causes, and prognosis depends on the cause, the severity of injury, and the duration of the state. Some patients recover; in others, a prolonged disorder of consciousness develops. The word "coma" alone can therefore never serve as the basis for an end-of-life decision. The cause, the examinations performed, the time that has passed, and the degree of certainty about the possibility of recovery must all be established.

In what is now often called unresponsive wakefulness syndrome, previously termed a "vegetative state," sleep-wake cycles may be present and the person may open the eyes, but there is no reliable behavioral evidence of awareness of self or environment. In a minimally conscious state, by contrast, there are limited but reproducible signs of awareness, such as visual tracking, appropriate responses, or non-random execution of a command. The distinction matters because it affects prognosis, rehabilitation, communication with the family, and assessment of the person's ability to participate in decisions.

The American Academy of Neurology guideline on prolonged disorders of consciousness, published in 2018 and reaffirmed in 2024, emphasizes systematic and repeated assessment rather than a diagnosis based on a brief encounter. Sedating medications, pain, infection, metabolic abnormalities, fatigue, and visual or hearing impairment can conceal responses. Nursing staff and family members may also identify a behavioral pattern that did not appear during a single examination. Their information is important, but it should enter an organized clinical process rather than turn every reflex movement into proof of awareness.

Consciousness, Communication, and Capacity Are Three Different Axes

The capacity to be conscious, the capacity to communicate, and the capacity to make a decision are not the same attribute. A person may be fully conscious yet unable to speak, for example because of motor paralysis or impairment of the muscles of speech. Another person may speak fluently yet be confused, delirious, or unable to understand the significance of the specific decision. Capacity must therefore not be inferred from outward appearance, and incapacity must not be inferred from disability.

ALS provides a clear example. Severe weakness can progress to loss of speech and independent breathing while mental clarity remains intact in many patients. A system that fails to provide alternative communication—an alphabet board, eye tracking, an adapted computer, or adequate time for a response—may in practice deprive a fully capable person of autonomy. Accessibility here is not an added convenience. It is a condition for law and ethics to recognize the person behind the disability.

Dementia can present the opposite picture. A person may walk, speak, laugh, and engage with others while gradually losing memory, judgment, and the ability to understand complex information. The question is then not whether the person is alive or communicating, but which decisions the person can still make and with what degree of support. A later chapter on dementia will examine the tension between earlier wishes and the person who is living in the present. For now, the medical principle is enough: a diagnosis of dementia does not automatically equal incapacity, and capacity is assessed in relation to the particular decision and at the time that decision is required.

Persistent, Prolonged, and Irreversible States

Words such as "permanent" and "irreversible" are sometimes used as though they express the same degree of certainty. They do not. Time alone does not make a diagnosis irreversible, and prognosis depends on the cause of the injury, age, clinical findings, and the course of recovery. In prolonged disorders of consciousness it may be necessary to revise a diagnosis after repeated assessments. Professionally, humility is not weakness: "we do not yet know" may be the correct answer, provided it is accompanied by a plan for investigation, rehabilitation, and reassessment.

This distinction has legal weight because irreversible decisions should rest on a degree of certainty proportionate to their seriousness. That does not mean that every treatment must continue until an absolute certainty—one that medicine may never be able to provide—has been reached. It means that the care team should distinguish clearly between what is known, what is estimated, and what cannot yet be known. Recording that distinction is more useful than a global statement such as "there is no chance," which does not explain what chance was assessed or on what evidence the assessment was based.

The Legal Meaning: Who Is Dead, Who Is Alive, and Who Can Decide

A determination of death fundamentally changes a person's legal status. Once brain-respiratory death has been determined according to law, the case is no longer that of a living patient refusing treatment or a dying patient governed by the Dying Patient Law. By contrast, a person in a coma, unresponsive wakefulness syndrome, a minimally conscious state, or a neurodegenerative condition is alive. The legal questions in such cases are who has authority to decide, what the person's wishes are, what benefit treatment is expected to provide, and what the law permits—not whether the person is already dead.

The distinction also protects against value judgments disguised as medical judgments. A neurological diagnosis describes function; it does not determine that a person's life has less value. A person who is completely dependent may still experience connection, pleasure, and meaning. Another person may define dependence as a condition he or she would not be willing to endure. Medicine must describe the state and the available options, and law must protect capacity and wishes, but neither may turn level of function into a measure of human worth.

A practical rule follows for the remainder of the book: before any end-of-life discussion, four questions should be separated—Is the person alive? What is the level of consciousness? Can the person communicate? Does the person have capacity to make this particular decision? Only after these axes have been distinguished can questions of treatment, autonomy, and avoidance of life prolongation be addressed responsibly.

Diagnosis, Trust, and Public Language

Neurological determinations do not exist only between professionals. A family may see a person who looks warm, whose heart is beating and whose chest rises and falls. The language used to explain a determination of brain-respiratory death is therefore almost as important as the protocol itself. A phrase such as "the brain has stopped working" may sound to a family like a very severe but potentially reversible condition. A precise explanation should make clear that the determination concerns complete and irreversible loss of brain functions under the criteria established by law, and that a ventilator can temporarily maintain bodily processes that do not change the determination of death.

Trust is also shaped by the way clinicians respond to questions and doubt. A family that asks who performed the tests, why an instrumental examination was required, and how the process relates to organ donation is not necessarily "opposed to medicine." Often it is trying to reconcile what it sees with its own eyes with a conclusion that is not intuitive. A transparent process, separation between determination of death and transplantation, and reasonable time for questions are part of professional quality, because a correct determination that is poorly explained can leave distrust for years.

Neurological Documentation as the Basis for Later Decisions

Even when the person is alive, accurate documentation of the state of consciousness is critical. General phrases such as "unresponsive," "vegetative," or "severe neurological condition" do not tell a later reader whether the person opened the eyes, visually tracked, followed commands, responded consistently to a familiar voice, or was receiving medication that reduced alertness. The more consequential the treatment decision, the more the medical record should allow a later reader to understand the diagnosis and degree of certainty on which it rested.

Such documentation is also important when the condition changes. A person may progress from coma to unresponsive wakefulness and later show signs of minimal consciousness. If all these changes are collapsed under one label, the team may continue a plan that no longer matches the patient's condition. Assessment of consciousness is therefore a process, not a stamp. It should be linked to a plan: when will the patient be reassessed, which findings would change the diagnosis, and when is another specialist opinion required?

Cardiac Arrest, "Clinical Death," and the Boundary Between a Reversible State and a Determination of Death

Public language sometimes uses the expression "clinical death" to describe cardiac arrest. Professionally, however, caution is required: a temporary cessation of pulse and breathing is not necessarily a determination of death if circulation can still be restored through resuscitation. This is precisely the distinction between an emergency state in which the duty to attempt rescue may be immediate and a determination of death after cessation of circulation and breathing has become irreversible according to professional criteria.

The distinction also matters when discussing do-not-resuscitate orders. A person who asks not to receive CPR is not "asking to be declared dead early"; the person is asking that one particular attempt to reverse cardiac arrest not be made. If cardiac arrest occurs and CPR is not performed in accordance with a valid instruction, death is determined after the condition meets the medical criteria. Refusal of a procedure and determination of death are two separate stages, and merging them under the expression "clinical death" can obscure the difference.

Even after successful resuscitation, return of a pulse is not the same as return of the person to the previous condition. Return of spontaneous circulation is an initial physiological goal, not a promise of neurological recovery. After prolonged cardiac arrest, severe brain injury may remain, and the discussion then shifts from whether to resuscitate to questions of prognosis, consciousness, and goals of care. The same event thus shows why end-of-life care cannot be evaluated by a single measure such as "we managed to restore a pulse."

Part Two

The History in Israel and the Road to the Dying Patient Law

Chapter 1

Decision-Making in Israel Before the Law: Physicians, Families, and the Courts

How End-of-Life Decisions Were Made in Israel Before the Law

Before 2005, Israel did not have a dedicated and comprehensive statutory framework for the dying patient. Decisions were made through a combination of general law, the Patients' Rights Law, case law, medical procedures, professional ethics, and local practice. This sometimes produced differences between institutions and teams and uncertainty about the limits of authority.

In practice, physicians and families had to decide whether to resuscitate, ventilate, continue cancer treatment, or undertake other interventions. When the patient had capacity and could express a wish, the right to refuse treatment carried weight through the principles of informed consent. The problem became more difficult when the patient lost capacity without leaving clear instructions.

Without a uniform mechanism for advance directives, families were sometimes asked to "decide" even when they did not know what the person would have wanted. Physicians worried about liability if treatment were stopped, while relatives feared that by agreeing not to continue they themselves were causing the death. Legal uncertainty therefore tended at times to make continued treatment the default.

This experience demonstrated that autonomy cannot rely solely on a conversation held in real time. A person who loses consciousness needs a mechanism that allows earlier wishes to continue to operate. That need became one of the central forces behind the future statutory arrangement.

Israel before the Dying Patient Law was not a legal vacuum. Decisions about resuscitation, ventilation, surgery, artificial nutrition, and the treatment of terminally ill patients were made every day through a combination of clinical judgment, informed consent, professional procedures, case law, and general legal principles. The difficulty was fragmentation. A physician in one department might rely on a local protocol; another family might turn to court; and in a dispute it was not always clear which principle should prevail. This lack of uniformity is one of the reasons a dedicated statute became necessary.

The traditional model of Israeli medicine, like that of other countries, was more paternalistic than the model common today. The physician was perceived as the holder of knowledge who decided what was best for the patient, and in some cases a difficult diagnosis was disclosed to the family before it was disclosed to the person concerned. Cultural and legal change, especially the strengthening of informed consent, challenged this structure. At the end of life the shift was particularly sensitive: moving from the medical question "what is right?" to the question "what would the patient want?" required not only legal reform but a change in habits of communication.

Even before the dedicated law, a patient with capacity was not a body that the medical system could treat as it wished. Principles of informed consent and bodily integrity limited treatment without consent. Yet when refusal was expected to result in death, professionals and families sometimes found it difficult to accept. The tension between a legal right and the medical instinct to save life produced cases in which legal clarification was sought. A dangerous refusal does not become invalid merely because it sounds "unreasonable" to the physician if the person has capacity and understands the consequences.

The problem was harder when patients lacked capacity. Without a clear statutory advance directive, the team had to learn from family members, prior conduct, and other documents what the person's wishes had been. Families acquired considerable practical power, but it was not always clear whether they were expressing the patient's wishes or their own distress. Relatives may ask to "do everything" out of guilt, or ask to stop out of exhaustion—not because they act in bad faith, but because they are human beings inside a crisis. The legal framework therefore needed a way to separate their voices from the patient's voice.

The absence of a dedicated law also made documentation of wishes less systematic. If a person had told a family physician years earlier that prolonged ventilation was not wanted, there was no guarantee that this information would reach an intensive care unit. Transitions between community care and hospital care could mean loss of information. A law that establishes forms and a registry seeks to solve exactly this problem: not merely to give legal force to wishes, but to make them accessible at the moment when the person can no longer express them again.

Clinically, physicians also had to decide when treatment was no longer beneficial. Law cannot require a physician to perform an intervention that lacks medical justification, but the boundary between a small chance and no chance is not always clear. Before the statute, some disputes reached legal advisers because a family requested treatment the team regarded as futile.

This created a tension that continues after legislation: autonomy confers the power to refuse, but does not necessarily create a right to demand every treatment.

Israeli society added a distinctive cultural layer. Memory of the Holocaust, wars, religious tradition, the value placed on saving life, and strong family ties contributed to reluctance toward decisions perceived as "giving up." At the same time, modern medicine and ideals of human rights strengthened demands for autonomy. The eventual Israeli compromise was therefore born not only between competing legal provisions but between different social stories about responsibility, family, and death.

Hospitals also developed local ethics mechanisms, but their availability and status were not uniform. A committee can assist when physicians and families disagree, yet without defined authority its capacity is limited. One of the purposes of dedicated legislation is to create a clearer address for disputes. Even so, no committee can substitute for early conversation. The more the system reaches a formal mechanism only after trust has broken down, the harder it is to reach a resolution the parties can accept.

The period before the law also teaches about defensive medicine. When a physician does not know whether stopping or not renewing treatment may create criminal or civil liability, continuing treatment can appear to be the safer choice. But "continuing" is not neutral for the patient; it can cause pain and prolong the process of dying. Legal certainty is intended not only to protect physicians from claims but also to protect patients from treatment given merely because nobody wants to bear the risk of making a decision.

From the perspective of medical negligence, this period illustrates how a standard of care can develop before a detailed statute exists. A physician still has duties to diagnose, explain, document, and treat symptoms according to professional standards. Ignoring a clear refusal or failing to treat pain does not cease to matter merely because there was no dedicated end-of-life statute. Later legislation adds a framework; it does not replace the basic duties of reasonable medical care.

Israel's pre-2005 history is therefore a history of partial solutions. Rights existed, judicial decisions existed, some physicians managed end-of-life care with sensitivity, and institutional mechanisms existed. What was missing was a single national language connecting medical definition, wishes, documents, palliative care, and the limits of permissible action. To understand why the law ultimately took the form it did, we must first examine who in practice held decision-making power: physicians, families, and courts.

The Law Does Not Begin with the Dedicated Statute

Before enactment of the Dying Patient Law, Israeli hospitals were still governed by the law of consent, duties of care, ethical principles, and case law. Decisions concerning resuscitation, ventilation, and continuation of treatment did not disappear; they were made within a less centralized framework. This is important because it shows that a dedicated statute does not create every right from nothing. It organizes and sharpens an existing normative system.

For lawyers, that point remains significant today. When the Dying Patient Law does not apply to a particular person, it does not follow that the person has no rights. The Patients' Rights Law, contract and tort law, constitutional principles, and professional rules may continue to apply. The legal question is therefore not only "does the special statute apply?" but also "which general framework applies if it does not?"

Institutionally, the pre-law period revealed variation. Physicians held different views, institutional committees did not operate in a single format, and families did not always know what options existed. Variation is not necessarily undesirable—medicine requires flexibility—but in irreversible decisions it can undermine equality and certainty. One aim of legislation was therefore to reduce dependence on the identity of a particular physician or institution.

History also helps explain why the statute contains detailed mechanisms. Requirements for documentation, authorized determination of status, advance documents, and committees are not accidental bureaucracy; they are responses to uncertainty exposed in practice. When considering reform, one should therefore ask what historical risk each mechanism was designed to address before abolishing or simplifying it.

What the Medical Record Teaches Us About the Pre-Law Period

From the perspective of medical law, the period before the statute demonstrates how a medical record can reveal culture. A chart may contain a brief sentence such as "the family agrees to no resuscitation," without documentation of any conversation with the patient, or an instruction such as "no aggressive treatment" without defining which interventions it includes. These are not merely technical omissions. They show how authority was understood at the time and why a more detailed mechanism became necessary.

From a nursing perspective, there could also be a gap between a general instruction and treatment during a shift. If the goal of care is not defined, a nurse facing falling oxygen saturation or a change in consciousness may summon a resuscitation team by default even though an earlier family discussion pointed in a different direction. Good law and good procedures must translate a value-based decision into clinical instructions that can be followed at two o'clock in the morning.

The central lesson is not that the system operated "without law," but that the duties were dispersed. Informed consent, the duty of care, reasonable treatment, and respect for human dignity already existed; later legislation connected them to a dedicated pathway. For the lawyer, the layers matter: even when a special provision does not apply, general law does not disappear.

The question of how decisions were made before the statute cannot be separated from the question of who in practice held the power to decide. Medical practice, the status of the family, and the gradual entry of courts into the field must therefore be examined together.

Physicians, Families, and the Courts: Who Made the Decision?

End-of-life decisions expose a tension among three centers of authority. The physician holds professional knowledge and can determine what is clinically possible and what lacks benefit. The family knows the person and may become that person's voice when communication is no longer possible. The court enters when a dispute cannot be resolved within the healthcare system.

None of the three has complete ownership of the decision. A family cannot demand medically unjustified treatment merely because it wants to "do everything." A physician cannot disregard the valid wish of a patient with capacity merely because the choice seems unwise. And a court, although empowered to decide disputes, cannot turn itself into a medical team.

Before the statute, cases that reached the courts demonstrated the need for a clearer framework. Courts had to consider refusal of treatment, capacity, the interests of an unconscious person, and the duties of the care team. Resort to litigation during the process of dying also revealed a practical limitation: legal proceedings are slow and heavy relative to clinical time. A sound system should therefore resolve most disagreements within healthcare and reserve the courts for exceptional cases.

This lesson influenced the creation of institutional committees and internal determination procedures in the future law. The aim was not to remove law from the hospital but to turn some legal principles into rules that could be implemented without calling a judge to every bedside.

In the classic model, physicians hold power through expertise. They know what a treatment can achieve, its risks, and the course of disease. Yet expertise does not tell them what a particular person considers a life worth living. When a physician decides alone that a treatment is "worth" the burden, fact and value are being mixed. The move toward shared medicine requires the physician to present the facts and give professional recommendations while leaving room for the patient's preferences where the law grants a choice.

The family holds another kind of power. It knows the person, remains present over time, and sometimes is the only source able to describe earlier wishes. But closeness is not immunity from error. Spouses and children may disagree, and the patient may have concealed preferences from them. Law therefore cannot assume that "the family" speaks with one voice. It is necessary to identify who has authority, who actually knows what, and who is expressing only a personal view.

Courts usually enter when other mechanisms fail. Their strength lies in external authority and the ability to interpret rights; their weakness lies in the fact that they operate more slowly than clinical reality and receive the case through documents and testimony. A judge does not stand at the bedside and observe changes from hour to hour. Access to a court is therefore an important tool, but not a routine solution for every treatment decision. A strong system resolves most cases within healthcare under clear rules and leaves courts for principled or exceptional disputes.

Before the statute, the relationship among these three centers of power was not always clearly defined. A physician might ask a family for "approval" of a do-not-resuscitate decision even when the patient was capable of deciding; a family might think it had a veto over the patient's wish; and a care team might turn to legal advisers when disagreement arose. Modern legislation seeks to order the hierarchy: first the capable patient, then the patient's earlier wishes when capacity is lost, and only afterward mechanisms of representation and adjudication.

Knowledge gaps influence the balance of power. A family may agree to continued treatment because it thinks the physician expects recovery, while the physician continues because he or she thinks the family is not ready to let go. Each side attributes to the other a wish that does not exist. A conversation in which the physician gives a clear recommendation—not merely a list of options—can prevent this loop of displaced responsibility. Shared medicine is not the transfer of the decision to the family; it is the combination of professional recommendation with the patient's wishes.

The medical team itself does not always speak with one voice. A senior physician, resident, nurse, and physiotherapist may see the patient differently. The nurse is at the bedside for hours and observes pain and agitation; the physician holds the diagnostic picture; rehabilitation professionals may identify functional potential. Good decision-making uses these differences rather than hiding them. A culture in which only the senior doctor's voice counts can lose important information.

Disputes over authority become more acute when the person lacks capacity and has left no document. The question then arises whether the decision should be based on "best interests" or on "substituted judgment." These are different tests. Substituted judgment seeks to reconstruct what the person would have chosen on the basis of his or her values; a best-interests approach asks what would benefit the person now. Sometimes the two converge; sometimes they do not. Legislation and case law need to clarify when each test is used so that the decision does not merely reflect the preferences of the person making it.

Family power also appears in the ability to resist transfer to hospice or to demand continuation of treatment. Sometimes resistance reflects misunderstanding of prognosis. If a physician says "we do not recommend further treatment" without explaining what care will still be provided, the family hears abandonment. Part of professional authority is the duty to communicate in a way that makes decision-making possible, not merely to determine clinically what is appropriate.

Legally, authority does not remove accountability. A person empowered to decide for another must act within the scope of that role; a physician exercising judgment must meet the standard of care; and an institution must create a process. When harm occurs, the legal question may not be who "decided to die," but whether the correct person made the decision on the basis of appropriate information and at the right time. That distinction is especially important in medical-negligence cases.

The period before the statute also showed that formal authority can differ from power in practice. A nurse without legal authority to discontinue treatment may have enormous influence on the conversation; a family member without a power of attorney may control access to the patient; an on-call physician may make a critical decision at night. Legal regulation must therefore connect to everyday work. If it exists only in the statute book, real power may remain elsewhere.

Case Law as the Place Where Facts Become Principles

End-of-life cases generally reach court after mechanisms of agreement have failed: relatives disagree, the care team and family are in conflict, or the patient cannot express a wish. Case law therefore often reflects difficult and exceptional situations rather than routine care. A researcher should be careful not to infer from the extreme case how the entire health system normally operates.

Yet exceptional cases are precisely the cases that generate principles. Courts are asked to define the weight of autonomy, evaluate evidence of earlier wishes, and decide the scope of professional authority. A judgment is also an evidentiary document: it reveals which facts were considered material, which expert opinions were submitted, and what information was missing. For a student of medical negligence, this makes case law an excellent source for learning how a medical record becomes legal evidence.

It is essential to distinguish legal doctrine from the facts of the case. A powerful sentence in a judgment may depend on narrow circumstances. Proper academic use requires reading the context, the remedy, and the precise question decided. A broad value statement should not be turned into an operational rule unless the court actually did so.

The limits of litigation must also be recognized. Courts are not always the best institution for rapid decisions while a patient is deteriorating. Proceedings are relatively expensive and slow, so a strong system tries to resolve most disagreements through communication, committees, and consultation, reserving judicial authority for cases in which a binding decision is necessary.

Authority Is Not a Substitute for Information

Debate over who has authority can distract from the question of what that person actually knows. A physician with medical authority who does not know the patient's values holds only half the picture. A relative who knows the person intimately but does not understand what resuscitation is likely to achieve holds the other half. A high-quality decision is created when clinical knowledge and personal knowledge meet within a clear structure of authority.

In a legal dispute, the chain of decision-making must be reconstructed: who communicated the prognosis, who took part in the conversation, whether the team gave a clear medical recommendation, and what legal status was held by the person speaking on the patient's behalf. Documentation stating only "spoke with family" is insufficient when several relatives held different views. The more irreversible the decision, the more important it is to identify precisely the authorized voice.

Nursing staff can serve as an early-warning mechanism when formal authority and reality drift apart. A nurse who notices that the patient is expressing a wish different from the one described by family members must know where and how to communicate that information. A professional culture that permits staff to raise doubt without treating it as an "end run" around the physician strengthens the safety of the decision.

This is why case law capable of defining limits and formulating principles became necessary. Israeli courts, even before the dedicated statute, encountered cases in which autonomy, the sanctity of life, and the patient's welfare came into conflict. The next chapter does not attempt to present every judgment in the field, but to identify the lines that developed and created the foundation for dedicated legislation.

Chapter 2

Israeli Case Law Before the Legislation

Israeli end-of-life case law developed against the background of Basic Law: Human Dignity and Liberty, the Patients' Rights Law, and criminal law. Courts recognized the tension between the sanctity of life and individual wishes and, in different cases, considered requests to withhold or discontinue treatment.

A central landmark in the period before the statute is CA 506/88 Yael Shefer v. State of Israel, PD 48(1) 87 (1993). The judgment concerned a request relating to the treatment of a child with Tay-Sachs disease and became a reference point in Israeli discussion of the sanctity of life, human dignity, and the boundary between withholding treatment and causing death. Its importance lies not in the idea that it alone "wrote" Israeli end-of-life law, but in the way it demonstrated how dependent judicial decisions are on the clinical facts and value framework of a particular case. The official background to the work of the Steinberg Committee likewise described pre-legislation case law as lacking uniformity and pointed to gaps between Shefer and some district-court decisions—one of the reasons a uniform statutory arrangement was sought.

One characteristic of the Israeli debate was the distinction between an active act causing death and refraining from prolonging life. This distinction is not unique to Israel, but it acquired particular weight at the meeting point of legal tradition, medical ethics, and Jewish law. The courts did not create a general permission for euthanasia, but they contributed to the understanding that a duty to protect life is not identical to a duty to impose treatment in every situation.

Cases involving severely ill patients also illustrated the difficulty of establishing wishes. A statement made to a relative, an earlier refusal of treatment, or a pattern of conduct over many years do not necessarily provide the same degree of certainty. This contributed to the need for a formal mechanism allowing a person to give instructions while healthy and capable.

Pre-legislation case law therefore functioned as a laboratory. It exposed the dilemmas, but could not by itself create a national system of forms, a registry, defined authorities, and statutory definitions. That role passed to the legislature.

Viewed cumulatively, the case law before the statute did not establish a general right to euthanasia and did not hold that every refusal of treatment automatically prevails. Its contribution was to establish limits: life is a central value, but it does not give the state or physicians unlimited authority over a person's body; conversely, autonomy does not necessarily create a right to demand that a professional intentionally cause death. This tension moved from the courts into the legislative process.

In medical law more broadly, informed-consent decisions strengthened the view of the patient as a participant rather than an object. The principle directly affects end-of-life care: if a person is entitled to decide about an operation that carries substantial risk, it is difficult to justify erasing that person's voice precisely when confronting terminal illness. Courts nonetheless had to examine capacity and understanding, because a refusal that may lead to death creates particular concern that the decision might be driven by a transient mental state or by a failure to appreciate the consequences.

Cases involving unconscious patients highlight the evidentiary problem. When no written instruction exists, every family statement about what "he always said" can be important, but must also be treated cautiously. A court may look for consistency, the circumstances in which statements were made, known values, and earlier conduct. The weaker the evidence, the greater the risk that the decision reflects the family rather than the person. Advance-directive legislation was intended in part to reduce reliance on retrospective reconstruction.

Case law also exposed the tension between acts and omissions. Criminal law tends to treat an act that causes death differently from a failure to continue treatment, yet in medical practice the line can be thin. If a treatment is stopped after it has begun, is that an act? If a device is programmed in advance to stop after a cycle, is failure to renew it an omission? Questions of this kind strengthened the need for a framework defining what may be done operationally rather than leaving clinicians with philosophy alone.

One of the central lessons of the cases is the importance of context. The same request has a different meaning when it comes from a person with capacity who speaks consistently than when it comes from a person with delirium; discontinuing an intervention has a different significance when the intervention is temporary than when every bodily function depends on it. Courts cannot choose one moral rule and apply it without facts. In medical cases, the clinical foundation—diagnosis, prognosis, alternatives, and wishes—is part of law, not merely background.

Israeli case law also developed within a constitutional framework that protects human dignity. Dignity can support protection of life, but it can also support the right not to be subjected to invasive treatment against one's wishes. This dual meaning contributed to the character of the later Israeli compromise. Rather than treat dignity as a single answer, the statutory arrangement would place it alongside sanctity of life and autonomy. That choice reflects a desire to acknowledge the value conflict rather than erase it.

For clinical staff, case law can become "law through stories." Physicians remember a famous case or headline and infer a rule from it. This can be dangerous. A judgment may be limited to its facts, may interpret the law that existed at the time, or may include a minority opinion. Institutional education should therefore translate case law into procedures rather than expect a nurse or an on-call physician to read judgments during a shift. The dedicated statute was designed to convert some of the principles into operational language.

The cases also demonstrated the limitations of the court as a medical institution. Litigation is adversarial: parties present arguments, experts are examined, and a judge decides. End-of-life care often requires a more collaborative and flexible process. Whenever a disagreement can be resolved through committee review, mediation, or conversation, it is generally preferable not to turn the bedside into an arena of litigation. The possibility of judicial review nevertheless remains essential when the institution itself is a party to the dispute or when basic rights are at risk.

From a medical-negligence perspective, these judgments also show that not every moral disagreement amounts to negligence. A physician may choose among several reasonable approaches and still reach a difficult outcome. Negligence requires deviation from a standard of care or breach of a legal duty. By contrast, treating a person contrary to a valid refusal, failing to disclose material information, or ignoring a treatable symptom can raise legal issues even when death itself was expected. The distinction between the outcome of the disease and the quality of the process is critical.

Pre-legislation case law remains important because it continues to operate through general legal principles that did not disappear in 2005. The Dying Patient Law is not a closed world. It coexists with the Patients' Rights Law, tort law, capacity and guardianship law, and constitutional principles. A lawyer or physician therefore cannot rely on a single statutory provision. The interaction among these frameworks must be understood.

The move from judicial decisions to legislation did not cancel the earlier law; it sought to organize it. Before turning to the Steinberg Committee, it is necessary to examine the statute that forms the background to almost every therapeutic relationship in Israel—the Patients' Rights Law—and why informed consent by itself was not enough to regulate end-of-life situations.

The Connection Between the Patients' Rights Law and End-of-Life Care

The Patients' Rights Law established in Israel principles of information, consent, privacy, and dignity within medical treatment. End-of-life decisions are an extreme test of those principles because a treatment decision may directly affect the length of life. Informed consent does not become less important when illness is severe; it becomes more complex because of emotional burden, uncertainty, and time pressure.

The right to refuse treatment is a central part of bodily autonomy, but its exercise requires capacity and information. The care team cannot simply record that "the patient refused" if it is unclear that the patient understood the significance of the decision. Conversely, a person must not be declared incapable merely because the choice differs from the physician's recommendation. This is the narrow line between protection and paternalism.

In medical negligence, a defect in consent may constitute a claim in its own right or may accompany a claim that the treatment itself was negligent. A procedure may have been performed competently but without disclosure of material information; alternatively, disclosure may have been adequate while the performance was defective. Separating these bases of liability permits a cleaner analysis.

The relationship to the Dying Patient Law illustrates the relationship between a general statute and a special statute. The dedicated end-of-life arrangement adds mechanisms for defined situations, but it does not abolish the culture of consent on which medical care is built. In fact, the earlier a patient participates in decisions through general patients' rights, the less the system will need to guess at that person's wishes after capacity is lost.

Case Law as a Way of Building a Clinical-Legal Language

End-of-life judgments are not only normative sources. They translate a medical event into legal questions: What is capacity? What constitutes a valid refusal? How should the wishes of a person who cannot communicate be established? What weight should be given to the risk of death? In this way, case law forces law to understand medicine and forces medicine to express its decisions in terms that can be reviewed.

Studying such a case requires reading beyond the bottom line. One must examine the patient's functional state, whether the intervention was temporary or prolonged, the prognosis, and what was said in real time. Two cases in which treatment was discontinued may be legally entirely different if one involved a clear refusal by a capable person while the other relied on a general evaluation of quality of life.

This is also where case law meets the law of negligence. A principled judgment defines rights, while a liability case examines whether the clinical team implemented them reasonably. Between the legal principle and the patient's bed lie details such as the timing of a conversation, documentation, assessment of capacity, and transfer of information between shifts. Those details are what allow a principle to live within a health system.

Chapter 3

From the Patients' Rights Law to the Steinberg Committee: The Need for a Dedicated Framework and the Israeli Compromise

The Tension Between the Patients' Rights Law and End-of-Life Questions

The Patients' Rights Law, 1996, was a milestone in Israel's transition from paternalistic medicine to a model that recognizes the patient as a rights-bearing person. Informed consent, privacy, information, and dignity received an explicit legal framework. Yet the statute did not fully answer the question of a patient who can no longer express a wish and is expected to die from an incurable disease.

The right to refuse treatment becomes especially difficult when refusal is expected to result in death. On the one hand, forcing treatment is a serious intrusion on the body and on autonomy. On the other, the clinical team has duties of rescue and care. When a person has decision-making capacity, the tension can often be resolved through that person's own choice. When capacity is absent, the law must answer who speaks on the patient's behalf and what evidence establishes the patient's wishes.

The Patients' Rights Law is also not the same as the Dying Patient Law. The former governs a broad range of therapeutic relationships; the latter is designed for a defined end-of-life situation and creates special mechanisms. That distinction matters because end-of-life directives must not be used incorrectly in circumstances that do not fall within the statutory definitions.

The later legislation did not replace the Patients' Rights Law. It added another layer. Its purpose was to give autonomy a form of continuing legal life even after a person loses the ability to speak, while preserving limits that the legislature considered essential.

The Patients' Rights Law produced a normative change by placing informed consent at the center of the therapeutic relationship. It requires disclosure of relevant information and recognizes that medical treatment is not justified merely because it is technically or professionally possible. At the end of life, that principle is especially important, but it does not solve every problem. A person may lack capacity; the situation may be urgent; treatment may already be under way; and the law must still determine which actions a physician may perform, withhold, or discontinue even when the patient requests a particular result.

Informed consent is a process, not a signature. A terminally ill patient who is handed a consent form in a language the patient does not understand has not been given meaningful autonomy. Refusal likewise requires information about its significance. When refusal may lead to death, the record should show that the person understood the expected consequences, the alternatives, and the possibility of changing his or her mind. The conversation need not become an interrogation, but it should demonstrate that the decision was informed.

The Patients' Rights Law also contains a framework for intervention in exceptional situations in which a person objects to treatment but special statutory conditions are present. These situations demonstrate that autonomy in Israeli law is not absolute. Yet an exception must not become a route for bypassing a patient's wishes simply because the care team finds them difficult to accept. Exceptions require defined conditions and careful interpretation, particularly when the person is lucid and consistent.

At the end of life, two distinct questions therefore collide: 'Has the patient consented to the treatment?' and 'Does the law permit the decision being requested?' A patient may refuse surgery, but cannot rely on informed consent doctrine to compel a physician to inject a lethal substance when the act is prohibited. The Patients' Rights Law structures the therapeutic relationship, while the Dying Patient Law adds end-of-life-specific limits. The distinction between a right to refuse and a right to demand is essential to understanding the two statutes together.

Privacy and confidentiality, also part of patients' rights, take on particular significance in the family setting. Physicians commonly speak with spouses and children, but a competent adult may ask that information not be shared. Approaching death does not cancel confidentiality. Conversely, if the patient wants family members involved, a team that excludes them may make implementation of decisions more difficult. The team should therefore clarify explicitly who may receive information and whom the patient wants present.

The right to information can also include, within the limits of law and circumstance, a wish not to receive some information. Some patients do not want numerical estimates or precise prognostic forecasts. Autonomy may include choosing to delegate parts of decision-making to a trusted relative. A system that forces every person to behave as an 'independent rational consumer' is not necessarily respectful. Even so, a wish not to know does not automatically authorize the family to decide without a legal and factual basis; the record should show how the person wanted information and decisions to be managed.

The link to medical negligence is especially clear in informed-consent cases. A claim may concern not technical performance, but the failure to disclose information that could have changed the decision. At the end of life, the possible harm may be treatment the person would have refused, a period of dependency, pain, or the loss of an opportunity to choose where to die. Causation can be complex: the question is what the person would have chosen if adequate information had been provided, not merely whether the treatment was medically successful.

The Patients' Rights Law also requires humane treatment and respect for dignity, principles that acquire practical content at the end of life. Privacy during bathing, the presence of family, prevention of pain, and respectful language are not optional additions to care. A person may have no prospect of cure and still possess full rights. That basic point prevents the label 'terminal' from becoming a category of reduced care.

The principal limitation of the Patients' Rights Law in this context is simply that it was not designed to answer every end-of-life question. By itself it does not create the detailed mechanism of advance medical directives for a dying patient, does not define the distinct Israeli treatment categories of continuous and cyclical treatment, and does not provide every special dispute-resolution mechanism. The need for another statute therefore does not show that the Patients' Rights Law failed; it shows that end-of-life care required an additional regulatory layer.

The relationship between the statutes also matters for interpretation. Rather than treating the Dying Patient Law as an exception that erases patients' rights, it is more accurate to understand it as a special arrangement operating within a legal culture of autonomy and dignity, while adding the value of sanctity of life and specific limitations. When uncertainty arises, the correct question is which issue each statute governs, not which one should replace the other.

This leads to the turning point. Israel already had patients' rights, case law, and medical practice, but it still needed a framework capable of formulating a workable compromise around end-of-life care. The Steinberg Committee was established for precisely that purpose, bringing together a broad group of physicians, lawyers, ethicists, religious scholars, and other representatives. Its composition itself demonstrated that the problem was never medical alone.

Why an Institutional Decision-Making Mechanism Was Needed

End-of-life disputes commonly combine facts, values, and relationships. A physician may believe that treatment is no longer beneficial; a family may believe that the physician is giving up too early; another professional may understand the prognosis differently. An institutional committee is meant to create a space in which the disagreement can be broken down and the true point of conflict identified.

A sound process begins with facts: diagnosis, prognosis, capacity, wishes, documents, and available treatments. Only then should the discussion move to values. Sometimes an apparently moral disagreement turns out to arise from a medical misunderstanding; sometimes the opposite occurs - everyone agrees on the facts but disagrees about the weight to assign to the competing values.

A multidisciplinary composition can reveal blind spots. A physician contributes clinical knowledge, a lawyer the normative framework, nursing and social-work professionals knowledge of function and family circumstances, and a public representative a perspective that is not purely institutional. Yet a large membership does not guarantee quality if the committee lacks time, information, or independence.

From the standpoint of responsibility, a committee decision is not immunity. If incorrect data were presented, or if the committee acted outside its authority, the process may still be subject to criticism. Its advantage lies in creating a reconstructable procedure: who was heard, what was considered, and what was decided. In complex cases, the existence of an orderly process may itself be important evidence of reasonable professional conduct.

Informed Consent at the End of Life Is Not a Form

At the end of life, the information that is material to a decision changes. A patient needs more than a list of procedural complications. The patient needs to understand how treatment is likely to affect the time remaining, the likelihood of returning home, the degree of dependency, and the chance of meaningful recovery. When such information is reasonably available but is not communicated, consent may be merely formal.

Refusal also requires professional work. Hearing 'I don't want it' and closing the file is no more sufficient than obtaining a signature on a consent form. The team should determine whether the person understands the meaning of refusal, whether a reversible condition is affecting the decision, and whether less burdensome alternatives have been offered. Respect for autonomy does not mean indifference to the process by which a choice is made.

From a nursing perspective, explanation does not end with one conversation. A patient may ask the same question again after the physician leaves or may express a fear that could not be voiced during a formal meeting. A nurse does not replace the physician in obtaining consent for a procedure, but can identify a gap in understanding and bring the issue back to the team. In this way, informed consent becomes an ongoing process rather than a single item of documentation.

The tension between the Patients' Rights Law and end-of-life questions demonstrated the need for a dedicated framework. The work of the Steinberg Committee was an attempt to transform that tension into a practical normative structure capable of functioning at the bedside.

Five Questions the Earlier Framework Did Not Resolve

The framework that preceded the Dying Patient Law left several fundamental questions without a sufficiently clear answer. The first was scope. Not every serious disease is an end-of-life condition, and not every patient with an incurable illness is at the same medical point. It was necessary to determine who enters the dedicated legal framework, who is authorized to make that determination, and how to deal with prognosis when certainty is impossible.

The second question was how to continue respecting a person's wishes after that person can no longer express them. The Patients' Rights Law strengthened informed consent, but end-of-life decisions are often required precisely after capacity has been lost. A mechanism was therefore needed that would allow a person to leave prior wishes in a form that could be authenticated and implemented, and to determine who may represent the person when no directive fully addresses the situation that has arisen.

The third question concerned the structure of the medical act. Is not starting a treatment equivalent to stopping a treatment that is already operating? Does it matter legally that a device functions continuously, while another treatment is given in separate cycles that require renewal? The question was not theoretical. It determined what a clinical team could do at the bedside without fearing that it had crossed the line between refraining from treatment and causing death.

The fourth question was affirmative rather than merely restrictive: what must the state offer a patient when the underlying disease cannot be cured? If legislation addressed only the prohibition on killing and permission to refrain from treatment, it would miss pain, dyspnea, anxiety, family support, and accompaniment. This was the reason palliative care had to become part of the legal arrangement rather than an optional addition provided by some institutions.

The fifth question was institutional: how can a serious disagreement be resolved quickly enough? End-of-life decisions may arise at night, in intensive care, or after sudden deterioration. A route that requires every case to reach a court is impractical, but a solitary decision by one professional may also be insufficient when a major dispute exists. The framework therefore needed an internal health-system procedure that combined documentation, transparency, and the possibility of review.

These were the problems that justified moving from a general patients' rights statute to a dedicated end-of-life framework. The public committee that followed did not have to invent the dilemmas; its task was to turn them into a single system of rules capable of being applied in different clinical situations. The structure of the committee, its method of work, and the way it sought consensus belong to the next stage of the story.

Chapter 4

The Birth of the Dying Patient Law and Its Fundamental Principles

The Enactment of the Law in 2005 and Its Background

The Dying Patient Law, 2005, emerged from a gap between the capabilities of modern medicine and the ability of the existing legal framework to provide consistent answers in end-of-life situations. Before its enactment, decision-makers could rely on general principles of informed consent, case law, ethics, and professional procedures, but there was no single system defining who qualifies as a dying patient, how wishes are established when capacity is absent, what legal status belongs to earlier instructions, and what limits bind the treating team.

The Israeli legislature did not choose a pathway built around a 'right to die.' Nor did it choose preservation of life at any cost. The statute is constructed as a balancing mechanism. Its starting point is that life has value, while a person's wishes and quality of life also have legal significance. This is not merely a philosophical declaration. It explains why the law permits refraining from certain forms of treatment while prohibiting acts whose direct purpose is to cause death.

The legislation was shaped by Jewish legal tradition, modern law, and clinical practice. The result was not a copy of the Dutch, American, or any other foreign model. It includes tools such as advance medical directives, powers of attorney, institutional committees, and the distinction between continuous and cyclical treatment. Some of these mechanisms are familiar elsewhere; their combination is, to a considerable extent, distinctly Israeli.

Enactment also conveyed an institutional message: end-of-life decisions should not remain in the gray area of 'this is how our department does it.' When a decision may determine whether treatment is provided or withheld, definitions, documentation, responsibility, and avenues of review matter. The law sought to reduce both unwanted treatment and uncontrolled decisions to limit treatment.

At the same time, a statutory framework does not guarantee meaningful use. Even at the time of enactment, it was clear that success would depend on public awareness, staff training, access to the required forms, and availability of palliative care. Implementation would later become one of the central points of criticism of the arrangement.

The Dying Patient Law was adopted in 2005 after years of public and professional debate. It entered a field already shaped by other legal principles. It did not repeal the Patients' Rights Law and did not replace the law of legal capacity. Rather, it created a special arrangement for situations in which incurable disease and limited life expectancy bring the question of life prolongation to the center. It should therefore be read as lex specialis in a defined field, not as a code governing every end-of-life medical decision.

The statute sought to transform a value-based compromise into a mechanism usable in practice. For that reason it contains not only declarations about sanctity of life and autonomy, but also definitions, methods for establishing wishes, documents, committees, treatment duties, and prohibitions. Structure matters. Reading only the principles section misses the way values are translated into action; reading only a form or administrative procedure loses the reasoning behind the framework.

A dedicated statute reduces some of the uncertainty faced by clinical staff. Before enactment, a physician might fear that not renewing treatment would be characterized as a criminal act or as negligence. A law that defines conditions creates a safer professional space. Legal certainty, however, is never absolute. Complex clinical situations do not always fit neatly into a provision, leaving room for interpretation, committee review, and legal advice.

The law also tries to protect against two opposite errors: prolonging life contrary to a valid wish, and withholding or discontinuing treatment without an adequate basis. It therefore requires examination of both the medical condition and the person's wishes. These are separate axes. A person may meet the medical definition and still want treatment; another may refuse treatment without falling within the statute's special framework. Professionals must know which law governs each axis.

One consequence of legislation is the creation of a new public vocabulary. Expressions such as 'dying patient,' 'advance medical directives,' and 'cyclical treatment' entered the language of end-of-life care. Yet legal terminology can remain inaccessible. If citizens do not know that the law exists, their practical ability to plan ahead is limited. The law's success therefore depends not only on enforcement but also on explanation and integration into routine care.

Israeli legislation did not permit active euthanasia. This point must be clear at the outset because confusion is common. The Dying Patient Law is not an 'euthanasia law' and does not create a route by which a physician may end a patient's life on request. It primarily regulates decisions regarding life-prolonging treatment and relief of suffering while maintaining a prohibition on acts intended to cause death.

The statute was enacted before some of the technological and social developments of the following two decades. Home-based medical care expanded, information systems improved, new therapies prolonged life in diseases that once had shorter courses, and international debate about assisted dying evolved. Contemporary reading must therefore distinguish stable principles from details that may warrant revision. The statute is not merely a historical text; it is a working tool that must function in a changing reality.

From the perspective of medical law, dedicated legislation sharpens the standard of care. When a statute prescribes a process, failure to follow it may have legal significance beyond the underlying clinical judgment. Technical compliance, however, is not always enough. A physician may complete the form but fail to explain; a health system may maintain a registry that nobody checks. Courts may therefore consider both the letter of a procedure and the broader duty to act as a reasonable professional.

The law also creates a direct interface between the state and deeply personal decisions. A person can deposit a document in a national registry and thereby ask the state to preserve that person's voice for the future. This is a distinctive use of public power: not to impose a decision, but to protect a decision from the loss of memory and information. The value of that mechanism depends on public trust that the document will be preserved, found when needed, and interpreted carefully.

The starting point for the chapters that follow is therefore that the statute is a system, not a single section. Its components include purpose, definitions, capacity, earlier wishes, powers of attorney, committees, treatment limits, and treatment categories. Once each component is explained in its proper place, later chapters can focus on how the components interact in real cases without repeating the entire statutory scheme each time.

Reading the Law as a System

The Dying Patient Law combines principles, definitions, methods for establishing wishes, treatment provisions, and dispute-resolution mechanisms. Professional reading should not begin and end with the particular section that happens to interest the reader. One must ask how the section depends on statutory definitions, what cumulative conditions are required, and what general legal rules continue to apply. In a field in which an error can affect life itself, systemic reading is part of safety.

For a law student, a useful method is to build a decision map for every case: scope; capacity; wishes; type of treatment; prohibitions; exceptions; authorized decision-maker; documentation; and dispute mechanism. Such a map prevents a leap to conclusions and helps separate medical questions - for example, prognosis - from legal questions such as who is authorized to make a determination or decision.

The statute should also be read together with regulations, forms, and administrative guidance. Statutory text may establish the principle while the daily operational details appear in a procedure. From the standpoint of responsibility, a professional cannot rely on a general memory of the law when an updated procedure that should have been known provides the relevant steps.

Medical Legislation as a System of Decisions, Not a Collection of Prohibitions

It is easy to read medical legislation through the question 'what is permitted and what is prohibited?' In practice, much of the statute's work occurs earlier: who gathers information, who may determine medical status, how wishes are preserved, which document is used, and when a committee should be approached. The quality of the legal arrangement is found largely in the process, not only at the final decision point.

For the clinical team, this means that an end-of-life decision must be transferable. A senior physician may understand the reasoning perfectly, but if the decision is not translated into the medical record and clear treatment orders, it may not survive a change of shift. The statute therefore creates an institutional responsibility not merely to reach the right decision, but to build a system in which the next person caring for the patient knows what was decided and why.

A dedicated law does not replace the reasonable-physician standard or the duty of reasonable nursing care. It adds another layer. A team can complete every required form and still fail to treat pain; it can provide clinically skilled care while ignoring a valid directive. Quality lies in connecting compliance with the legal norm to sound clinical practice.

The background to the legislation explains why the law did not settle for one prohibition or one permission. The disputes that preceded enactment produced a set of fundamental principles intended to guide decisions before any specific provision is applied.

The Purpose of the Law and Its Fundamental Principles

The law seeks to regulate medical treatment of a dying patient by balancing three centers of concern: the value of sanctity of life, the autonomous wishes of the person, and the significance of quality of life. Writing the three together is important. The legislature does not assume that autonomy erases sanctity of life, nor that sanctity of life eliminates personal wishes.

The first principle is a presumption in favor of the will to live. The law starts from the premise that life should be protected unless a different wish has been established with sufficient reliability through a mechanism recognized by law. The presumption protects the patient in situations of uncertainty, particularly when the person cannot speak. It guards against easy assumptions by relatives or institutions that a person 'would not want to live like this' without reliable evidence.

The second principle is recognition of expressed wishes. When a person with capacity states a position regarding treatment, that position carries central weight. When capacity is lost, the law provides a hierarchy of evidence, including advance medical directives, a power of attorney, and other sources recognized by law. In this way, the statute attempts to extend autonomy from the present into the future.

The third principle is that certain acts remain prohibited even when requested by the patient. The law does not permit active euthanasia and does not authorize assistance in suicide. This places a limit on autonomy: a person may request that certain interventions not be performed, but the statute does not create a claim to receive an act whose direct purpose is to cause death.

The fourth principle is non-abandonment. A decision not to provide life-prolonging treatment does not release the health system from duties of palliative, nursing, and supportive care. This is critical to the statutory design. The aim is not a pathway to 'less care,' but a distinction between treatment that prolongs the process of dying and treatment that relieves suffering.

The fifth principle is procedure. Determining medical status, establishing wishes, and documenting the process are not technical details. When a patient lacks capacity, the process itself becomes part of the protection of that person. Poor documentation can make even a clinically sound decision difficult to defend after the fact.

Purpose and principles sections are not literary prefaces. They guide interpretation when a specific statutory provision is ambiguous. In the Dying Patient Law, the balance among sanctity of life, autonomy, and quality of life is a deliberate statement that the legislature did not adopt any one value as absolute. An interpretation that completely erases personal wishes in the name of life, or one that ignores every limitation in the name of autonomy, is difficult to reconcile with the structure of the law.

Sanctity of life in the statute is not necessarily identical to a religious doctrine. It also operates as a public principle protecting against devaluation of human life because of age, disability, dependency, or cost. It helps explain why the statute does not permit intentional killing. Yet the same statute recognizes that protecting life does not always require prolonging the dying process by every available technology. The value of life is therefore distinct from a duty to use every possible means.

Autonomy is expressed through the patient's wishes, but it is not exercised in a vacuum. The statute asks whether the person has capacity, whether a directive is valid, and whether the present situation falls within its terms. It also limits certain acts that a person may request. This is autonomy within a framework, not absolute ownership. The arrangement reflects the view that the state must respect choice broadly while remaining entitled to define limits on the kinds of acts professionals may perform.

Quality of life is the most sensitive principle because it can easily become an external judgment. The statute should not authorize a physician to decide that the life of a person with a disability is of 'low quality' and therefore less worthy of protection. The relevant question is how the person experiences the burdens involved and what the goals of treatment are. Quality of life may provide clinical and personal information, but it must never become a ranking of human worth.

The principle of relief of suffering gives the law a positive dimension. The arrangement does not merely permit refraining from treatment; it requires continued care. Pain, dyspnea, anxiety, secretions, and nursing needs remain within the sphere of responsibility. This also protects against a situation in which a person 'chooses' aggressive treatment only because the alternative offered is abandonment.

The principles also shape the treatment of uncertainty. When the meaning of an old directive is unclear, respect for autonomy requires a genuine attempt to reconstruct the person's wishes, while the value of life warns against expansive interpretation of weak evidence. When a treatment no longer offers reasonable medical benefit, the goals of avoiding prolonged dying and relieving suffering gain weight. There is no mechanical formula, which is why the process must show how the competing considerations were evaluated.

For legal education, it is important to understand that balance does not mean finding a midpoint in every case. Sometimes autonomy clearly controls, as when a capable patient refuses a treatment the law permits that person to refuse. At other times an absolute prohibition on a particular act determines the result even when the wish is clear. 'Balance' describes the structure of the statute as a whole, not a license for a judge or physician to invent a new midpoint in every individual case.

The principles also explain the existence of oversight mechanisms. If the statute were based on wishes alone, a declaration would be enough. If it were based on life alone, a prohibition would be enough. Combining the values requires factual inquiry: Is the request authentic? Does the medical situation fit the statutory conditions? Is there a document, and what does it mean? Procedure is not accidental bureaucracy; it is the means by which the balance becomes operational.

For the public, the principles can be translated into simple language: the law does not require a person to accept every treatment, but it also does not permit a physician to cause death; it seeks to ensure that the person's wishes are clear and that suffering is treated. Such translation is often more useful than quotation of a statutory section. Citizens need to understand what they can do today to influence future treatment, not merely what values the legislature has announced.

In the chapters that follow, these principles will function as a compass rather than being redefined each time. The next question is when the statute is activated at all. That is the definition of a 'dying patient,' in which medical judgment becomes the gateway to legal rights and mechanisms.

The Balance Is Found in the Details

A declaration about sanctity of life, autonomy, and quality of life gives the statute direction, but it is not by itself a decision tool. The balance appears in the details: which acts remain prohibited even at the patient's request; when treatment may be withheld; how earlier wishes are proved; who may serve as an attorney-in-fact; and what role the committees play. Each mechanism gives weight to one value while simultaneously limiting it.

Criticism of the statute should therefore be concrete. Saying that it is 'too paternalistic' or 'too liberal' is not enough. Serious reform analysis identifies the provision or mechanism producing the result and proposes a plausible alternative. This makes discussion of reform more precise and prevents debate from being reduced to labels.

The same balance shapes clinical practice. A physician is not expected to resolve a philosophical controversy personally, but to act within a legal and professional framework. When the framework is unclear, appropriate consultation should be used rather than an improvised private compromise. In this way, the law converts a value conflict into rules of work that can be taught and reviewed.

Three Values When They Meet a Real Person

Sanctity of life, autonomy, and quality of life appear balanced on paper, but at the bedside they do not carry equal force at every moment. When a patient with capacity refuses an intervention, autonomy is at the foreground. When nothing is known about the person's wishes, protection of life gains greater weight. When treatment cannot cure and produces substantial suffering, relief becomes central. The law therefore requires not merely knowledge of the values, but the ability to recognize which one is most relevant to the particular type of decision.

Clinically, 'quality of life' is not a score assigned by the physician. It is made up of function, symptoms, and personal meaning. A patient willing to live with a tracheostomy in order to meet a new grandchild values that outcome differently from a patient who regards complete dependency as unacceptable. The team's role is to provide reliable information, not to substitute its own value system for that of the person.

Legally, good balancing can often be identified through reasoning. When the record shows the medical situation, the patient's wishes, the alternatives considered, and why a particular course was selected, the decision can be evaluated. When the chart says only 'supportive care decided,' the value-based work remains hidden. Reason-giving is not merely documentation for litigation; it is a tool that forces the team to think.

A Practical Decision Map: From Diagnosis to Decision

1. Establish the medical condition and prognosis and ask whether the statutory conditions are met, without turning medical uncertainty into artificial certainty.

2. Assess decision-making capacity in relation to the decision at issue. If the patient has capacity, the current wishes are the starting point; if capacity is absent, the process moves to earlier wishes and authority to represent the patient.

3. Locate advance medical directives, powers of attorney, and earlier documentation, and determine whether they are valid and relevant to the current clinical scenario.

4. Define the goal of treatment and classify the intervention: life-saving or life-prolonging treatment, palliative treatment, continuous or cyclical treatment, and whether the issue is withholding or discontinuation.

5. Document the information, the professional recommendation, the patient's wishes, and the alternatives. When a material disagreement or unresolved uncertainty remains, use consultation and the institutional committee as appropriate.

6. Translate the decision into clear treatment orders, communicate it across shifts and settings, and determine when reassessment is required if the condition, wishes, or goals of care change.

Chapter 5

The Steinberg Committee: Its Structure and the Path to Consensus

On February 20, 2000, the appointment of Professor Avraham Steinberg as chair of the governmental-public committee on the dying patient took effect. The Minister of Health at the time, Shlomo Benizri, charged the committee with preparing the foundation for legislation in an area in which case law, ethics, and medical practice had not produced a uniform rule. The committee had 59 members, and its unusually broad composition was part of the method: professional and value-based groups were to be represented before a legislative recommendation was formulated, rather than being asked merely to react to a bill already drafted by one discipline.

The work was divided among four subcommittees. The medical-scientific subcommittee, chaired by Professor Charles Sprung, included 26 physicians, nurses, and social workers; the philosophical-ethical subcommittee, chaired by Professor Asa Kasher, included 12 philosophers, ethicists, and religious scholars; the legal subcommittee, chaired by Professor Amnon Carmi, included 13 judges, jurists, and attorneys; and the halakhic subcommittee, chaired by Rabbi Yaakov Ariel, included seven experts in Jewish law drawn from the rabbinic and medical worlds. The division allowed each field first to formulate its difficulties in its own language and only then to examine whether the positions could be integrated into one legal arrangement.

The structure did not mean that each group possessed a veto over every detail. The discussions were meant to reveal where disagreements were factual, where they were linguistic, and where they were genuinely normative. A physician might speak about non-beneficial treatment, a lawyer about the limits of liability, a halakhic scholar about causing death or removing an impediment to dying, and a philosopher about autonomy. Different terminology can create the appearance of deep conflict even when the participants are describing the same situation from different angles. One purpose of the committee was therefore to create a shared language.

According to the official documents, the committee worked for almost two years. Despite intense disagreements, consensus was reached on five central principles: prohibition of active euthanasia; the possibility, under defined conditions, of refraining from treatment that delays death; a duty to provide palliative care; a transparent and orderly deliberative process in which the patient or a person representing the patient's wishes is heard; and recognition of the possibility of giving legal effect to advance medical directives. The significance of the consensus was the creation of common ground, not the elimination of every disagreement about implementation.

The committee illustrates an important lesson about policy-making in a sensitive field. Broad agreement does not require every participant to adopt the same philosophy. One person may place sanctity of life at the center, another autonomy, yet both may still agree on a mechanism that prohibits active euthanasia, respects a defined refusal, requires treatment of suffering, and provides a path for resolving disputes. This is compromise in an institutional sense - not abandonment of values, but construction of rules that allow them to operate together.

On January 17, 2002, the committee's report and proposed bill were submitted to Minister of Health Nissim Dahan. The discussion then moved from the professional-public arena into the governmental and parliamentary arenas. A committee can recommend and formulate consensus, but only the legislature can transform recommendations into binding rights, duties, and prohibitions. The next question was which recommendations would survive the legislative process and how they would be translated into provisions that could be implemented throughout the health system.

Chapter 6

From the Committee Report to the Knesset: The 2005 Decision

Submission of the committee report did not automatically turn its recommendations into law. Between 2002 and 2005, the subject went through governmental and parliamentary processing, during which the legislature had to decide details that could not remain at the level of general value statements. A government bill was laid before the Knesset in 2004, followed by deliberations in the Labor, Welfare and Health Committee as the legislation moved toward completion.

The debates were not centered only on the symbolic question whether Israel was 'for' or 'against' euthanasia. The legislature had to define terms that clinicians and institutions could actually use: what counts as an incurable illness; how life expectancy is assessed; who is the responsible physician; how capacity is determined; what weight belongs to an advance directive; what happens when no document exists; how minors are treated; and what route applies when the relevant parties disagree. Each definition can change the outcome of a particular case and is therefore part of the value judgment itself, not a merely technical matter.

A particularly sensitive issue was the distinction between not starting treatment and stopping treatment that has already begun. The Knesset had to translate the compromise created in professional discussions into a legal structure that clinical staff could recognize in real time. This produced detailed distinctions between continuous and cyclical treatment, between an act intended to cause death and refraining from prolongation, and between life-prolonging treatment and treatment whose purpose is relief of suffering. These are examples of legal drafting becoming a clinical instruction.

At the same time, the legislature sought to prevent the patient's wishes from remaining an abstract idea. Mechanisms were therefore created for advance medical directives, powers of attorney, an information registry, and decision-making committees. The choice of a system containing multiple mechanisms reflected the understanding that end-of-life care is not a single type of event. A capable person refusing treatment, a person who has lost capacity but left a document, and a person about whom no prior information exists present different questions and require different levels of verification and protection.

On December 6, 2005, the Dying Patient Law, 2005, was passed on second and third readings. It was published in the Book of Laws on December 15, 2005, and was scheduled to enter into force one year later, on December 15, 2006. The period before commencement had practical importance: the health system had to prepare forms, procedures, a registry, committee mechanisms, and training. A statute of this kind cannot be implemented merely by publication in the official gazette.

Historically, the 2005 decision marks the point at which the state accepted responsibility for replacing ad hoc decisions with a single normative system. The statute was designed to guide decisions before conflict arises while also enabling review when decisions are difficult. From this point, the discussion can move from how the law was created to how it works in practice: who falls within its definitions, how wishes are determined, and what the clinical team does when facts and values do not all point in the same direction.

Part Three

Israel After the Legislation: The Law in Practice, the Disputes, and the Person Behind Them

Chapter 1

Who Is a Dying Patient Under the Law?

The medical meaning of the terms 'terminal' and 'dying patient' was discussed in the conceptual part of the book. The focus here is narrower: when does the statutory definition that activates the mechanisms of the Dying Patient Law apply, who makes that determination, and how should it be documented so that it can function in real time?

The statute does not apply to every person with a chronic or incurable disease. It creates a definition linked both to the nature of the illness and to an assessment of life expectancy. In practical terms, a person with a severe disease may have a clear wish to avoid a particular treatment, but the special mechanisms of the Dying Patient Law operate only when the statutory conditions are met.

It is essential to distinguish the scope of the Dying Patient Law from the patient's general rights. A person who does not yet fall within the statutory definition does not thereby lose the rights of informed consent or the possibility of refusing treatment under general law. Conversely, satisfying the definition does not make every treatment unwanted. The law's applicability and the patient's wishes are two separate axes that must be examined independently.

The determination is made by a 'responsible physician' as defined by the statute and its procedures. In a medical institution, specified medical officeholders are authorized to make the determination; corresponding arrangements exist in community care. It is not enough for the patient or family to describe the person as terminal. The law thereby seeks to prevent self-activation of mechanisms that may have irreversible consequences.

Assessment of life expectancy requires clinical judgment. Medicine is not a clock. Some patients live substantially longer than predicted and others deteriorate more quickly. Prognosis should therefore be understood as a decision-making tool based on current medical knowledge, not as a promise. In diseases that do not progress along a straight line, such as heart failure or chronic lung disease, the determination is especially complex.

For a prognostic assessment to be reviewable, it is not enough to write 'life expectancy up to six months.' The record should identify the data on which the assessment rests: stage of disease, rate of deterioration, response to treatment, functional state, organ failures, and expected complications. Such documentation does not turn prognosis into certainty; it allows later readers to understand why the assessment was reasonable at the time.

The statute also distinguishes a stage closer to death, in which the medically estimated time remaining is very short. That distinction is relevant to some treatments and to the way the patient's wishes are implemented. The closer death becomes, the more acute the proportionality question surrounding aggressive interventions may be.

A sound legal definition must be rigid enough to prevent arbitrary use and flexible enough to reflect clinical reality. This tension is built into the subject. Israel chose to link the framework to prognosis; some foreign models use different criteria. The comparative chapters later in the book will show the costs and advantages of each approach.

A determination made too early can lead the team and family to interpret every treatment as 'pointless.' A determination made too late can deprive the person of time for planning and advance directives. The goal is not to attach a label but to activate a mechanism appropriate to the stage of illness. For that reason, physicians should not postpone discussion of end-of-life care merely because prognosis remains uncertain. Planning can begin before the formal legal status is established.

Israeli law also distinguishes stages within the end of life, and in practice it matters when life expectancy has become especially short. As death approaches, goals of treatment may change and the legal treatment of some interventions takes on a different context. Yet a time window must never become an automatic switch. A person may still want treatment at an advanced stage, and the statute is constructed around that person's wishes within the legal boundaries.

The determination must reach the people who need to act on it. If a senior physician establishes the status but it is not documented or transmitted across shifts, the team may continue full treatment by default. The medical record must be clear, and the organization must know where the determination appears. Here law meets information management: a right that is not visible on the relevant screen during an emergency may not protect the patient in practice.

Disagreement about prognosis may justify a second opinion. A family may present a specialist who sees a better chance of recovery; members of the treating team may disagree among themselves. A sound mechanism does not treat a second opinion as a threat but as a tool for testing a decision. In unusual cases, an institutional committee may assist. The objective is not to eliminate every uncertainty, but to ensure that the determination is not arbitrary.

From a tort-law perspective, an error in defining the patient's status can be significant if it leads to treatment contrary to the patient's wishes or to failure to treat a reversible problem. But an incorrect prognosis is not, by itself, necessarily negligence. The relevant question is whether the assessment met a reasonable professional standard on the basis of the information available at the time. Hindsight is not a substitute for examining the actual decision-making process.

For a lawyer, committee, or quality-review body examining the decision later, the timeline matters as much as the outcome: when did the prognosis change, who established the status, what information was available, whether a reversible problem was considered, and whether another opinion was needed. A later statement that 'the patient was terminal' cannot replace the clinical basis documented in real time.

The status should also be explained to the person. The sentence 'the law defines you as a dying patient' can be frightening if it is not accompanied by explanation. The patient should be told what the status means: which planning options become available, which treatments continue, who will make decisions, and what rights apply. The legal definition should become a tool that increases control, not a label that diminishes hope.

Once the statute is found to apply, the next question is who makes the decision. The starting point when a patient has capacity is entirely different from the position after capacity is lost. The following chapter therefore turns to the person who can understand and decide, and to the legally binding limits of that person's wishes.

Chapter 2

Capacity and Incapacity: How the Patient's Wishes Are Determined

A Patient With Capacity: How Far Must the Team Respect the Patient's Wishes?

When a patient has decision-making capacity, the starting point is that the patient is the central person in decisions about his or her own body. Capacity in this context is not the same as intelligence, education, or agreement with the physician. It concerns the ability to understand relevant information, appreciate its significance in relation to one's own condition, weigh alternatives in a reasoned way, and communicate a consistent choice.

A physician may believe that the patient's decision is dangerous or mistaken. That alone does not establish incapacity. A person is entitled to assign different weight to values than the physician does. One patient may prefer quality of life over prolongation, while another may prefer the opposite. The team's role is to ensure that the choice rests on information and understanding, not to replace the patient's values with its own.

A request, however, is not always binding. A patient cannot compel a physician to provide treatment that lacks medical justification, nor can the patient demand an act that the law prohibits. This is the distinction between a right to refuse and a right to demand. The right of refusal protects the boundaries of the body; a right to demand an act would impose an obligation on another person and on a professional system.

When a patient refuses life-prolonging treatment, a structured conversation is important: what does the patient understand about the condition, what is expected to happen without the treatment, are alternatives available, and what is the reason for refusing? Sometimes a request to 'stop everything' arises from pain or anxiety that can be treated. Addressing the cause may change the patient's wishes without undermining autonomy.

Assessment of capacity must also be sensitive to communication. Speech impairment, deafness, paralysis, or a language barrier does not amount to loss of capacity. The system must adapt communication methods so that the person can express a choice. Otherwise, a communication disability can mistakenly become a denial of rights.

A patient with capacity is the primary source of information about his or her wishes. The law does not require the family to approve the patient's decision, and family closeness does not create a veto. This point is important for teams to understand: in an effort to avoid conflict, clinicians may invite the children into the discussion and negotiate over a decision that already belongs to the patient. Family members may support and participate according to the patient's wishes, but they do not replace the patient.

Assessing capacity may be straightforward when a person is clear and alert, but it can be difficult in delirium, under the influence of medications, in dementia, or during severe distress. Capacity may also fluctuate during the day. It may therefore be appropriate to postpone a non-urgent decision until the person is more alert, treat a reversible cause, or involve a specialist. The objective is not to find a reason to deny capacity, but to create conditions in which the person can decide whenever possible.

A patient with capacity may also change his or her mind. A prior directive does not bind a person who can now decide. If the patient previously wrote that mechanical ventilation would not be wanted but, in the current situation, asks for a short trial, the current wish is the central consideration under the law. Documents are meant to speak when the person cannot, not to compete with the person when he or she can.

A physician must provide material information without overwhelming the patient. Prognosis, benefit, burden, and alternatives should be presented in language adapted to the person. A teach-back question - asking the patient to explain in his or her own words what was understood - can be a useful tool without turning the conversation into an examination. It reveals gaps while there is still time to correct them.

Genuine consent also requires freedom from pressure. Pressure may come from family members, a primary caregiver, financial constraints, or a sense of guilt. There is no need to assume in advance that relatives are acting improperly, but when an irreversible decision is made in the setting of deep dependency it is appropriate to offer the patient a private conversation as well. Sometimes only in a quiet room, without someone speaking on the patient's behalf, can clinicians learn what the patient actually wants.

Depression requires a precise approach. A psychiatric diagnosis does not automatically negate capacity, but severe depression can affect hope, judgment, and a wish to die. When an irreversible request appears alongside concerning signs, an appropriate evaluation is part of protecting the person's will. Psychiatry should not be used to invalidate every refusal, but neither should a treatable condition be ignored.

From a legal perspective, documentation of a conversation with a patient who has capacity should show the substance of the decision. There is no need to transcribe every sentence, but the record should identify the information given, the central questions discussed, the patient's wish, and the assessment of capacity when there is reason to document it. A note stating only 'the patient refuses' may be weak if a dispute later arises. Conversely, excessive template documentation that does not reflect a real conversation is not helpful.

The patient with capacity is the relatively simple case in terms of the source of authority, even when the decision itself is difficult. Once capacity is lost, the source of information changes: prior wishes must be investigated through the tools recognized by law. The remainder of this chapter therefore moves from the patient who can decide now to the way the wishes of a person who can no longer make a real-time decision are determined.

When the patient has capacity, the patient's wishes are heard directly. Loss of capacity changes the source of information, but it does not eliminate the need to determine the patient's wishes; it shifts the inquiry to documents, testimony, and the mechanisms established by law.

A Patient Without Capacity: How Are the Patient's Wishes Determined?

When a person can no longer make decisions, the risks of paternalism and guesswork increase. The law attempts to address this by moving from the question 'What does the family want?' to the question 'What would the patient want?' The distinction is fundamental. A relative or proxy does not own the person's life; the role is to represent the patient's wishes within the framework established by law.

Advance medical directives are the most direct evidence of prior wishes when they are valid and relevant to the situation that has arisen. A power of attorney allows a person to choose in advance who will act on his or her behalf, and when no such document exists it may be necessary to consider other evidence of the patient's wishes and preferences in accordance with the legal framework. The more explicit the evidence, the closer it is to the present decision, and the more consistent it is with the person's pattern of life, the easier it is to give it weight. The purpose is not to count relatives' votes, but to reconstruct the patient's own wishes as faithfully as possible.

Difficulty arises when a directive is old, general, or does not precisely fit the present situation. A person may have written that he or she does not want 'machines,' while the current treatment is temporary and offers a good chance of recovery. Is this the situation the person meant? Interpreting an advance directive requires understanding the values behind it rather than reading a single word in isolation.

A further conflict arises when the person now appears calm or content even though he or she previously wrote that life in a similar condition would not be wanted. The problem is especially sharp in advanced dementia: does the earlier person, who wrote the document from a particular understanding of life, bind the current person who can no longer understand the directive? Israeli law is not structured as a model of euthanasia pursuant to an advance directive, so the question concerns treatment decisions rather than a direct act intended to cause death.

Professionally and legally, the more vulnerable the patient, the more important it is to document the process by which the patient's wishes were determined. The record should show not only what was decided, but what the sources of information were, who participated, what authority each participant had, which documents were reviewed, which alternatives were discussed, and why a particular course was chosen. Such documentation protects against the possibility that system convenience, family exhaustion, or the most dominant relative unintentionally replaces the person's voice, and it allows changing teams to continue along the same reasoned course.

When there is no document, oral evidence becomes important. Statements the person made during the illness, views expressed about another relative's situation, lifestyle, and previous decisions may all help. A momentary statement such as 'I don't want to live like this,' made during severe pain, should be distinguished from a consistent position. A sound process gathers several sources rather than relying on the most dominant relative.

The current preferences of a person with partial ability are also information. Loss of capacity for a complex decision does not mean that the person has no wishes. A person with dementia may express fear, comfort, resistance to touch, or a preference for a particular person. The patient's voice should be respected as far as possible, and professionals should not speak about the person as if he or she were absent. Legal capacity and human participation are not the same thing.

The patient's best interests enter the picture when wishes cannot be determined. Best interests are not a test of convenience for the system. Pain, benefit, chance of recovery, burden, and alternative care must be considered. An assessment of 'quality of life' must be careful not to reproduce bias. A dependent person is not necessarily suffering, and an independent person may suffer greatly. When the person's wishes are unknown, the decision must be individualized and protected from stereotypes.

The family needs support because the representative role can be burdensome. A relative may feel that he or she is 'killing' the patient by respecting a directive not to continue treatment. A team that explains that the disease is the cause of death and that the family's role is to represent the person can reduce guilt. Sometimes that conversation is as important as the medical decision itself.

A conflict of interest does not necessarily imply bad faith. A relative may be troubled by expenses, inheritance, exhaustion, or emotional distress. There is no reason to suspect every family member, but when signs appear that a request is disconnected from the patient's wishes, further review is required. A committee or outside professional can assist. Protecting vulnerable people depends on the ability to pause a process when interests conflict.

Loss of capacity is the central reason the law created tools for advance planning. Instead of hoping that the family will remember, a person can deposit directives or appoint a proxy. The two tools are different: one gives instructions, the other gives another person authority to act. The following chapters distinguish between them.

Brief Case: Capacity Is Not Agreement With the Team

A patient with advanced disease refuses mechanical ventilation, understands that the refusal may shorten life, and explains consistently why the outcome of ventilation would be unacceptable. The family believes the patient is 'giving up.' The case illustrates that the question is not whether the decision appears correct to the team or the family, but whether the patient understands the information, appreciates its meaning, and chooses without an influence that negates the ability to decide. If delirium, uncontrolled pain, or unusual fluctuation appears, those problems should be treated and capacity reassessed - not presumed absent merely because the patient refuses treatment.

Chapter 3

Expressing Wishes in Advance: Advance Medical Directives and Power of Attorney

Advance Medical Directives

An advance medical directive is an attempt to bridge a gap in time. A person who has capacity states today what he or she would want done in the future if later defined as a dying patient and no longer able to express a decision. In this way the person attempts to preserve his or her voice beyond the loss of capacity.

As of August 2026, the Israeli Ministry of Health operates an online service and a national registry for advance medical directives and powers of attorney. According to the updated official information, a person aged seventeen or older who has capacity may issue directives or appoint a proxy. The documents become operative when the person has been defined as a dying patient and lacks capacity, and their validity is five years unless they are updated, extended, or revoked. The full procedures require professional explanation and signatures before witnesses in accordance with the relevant form, and a document deposited in the registry can be made available to authorized teams when needed. Because operational requirements may change, this book directs readers to the Ministry of Health's official service before actually completing the forms.

Israel has official forms and a dedicated Ministry of Health registry. The process includes medical explanation and details intended to ensure that the directive is not a general slogan but a decision based on an understanding of clinical situations and treatments. The document is time-limited and may be renewed or revoked, reflecting the principle that values and preferences can change over the course of life.

The form's advantage is also its weakness. The more detailed it is, the more precise it can be, but it may also become complicated and discouraging. A healthy person may find it difficult to imagine future clinical states. Terms such as ventilation, dialysis, artificial nutrition, or resuscitation are not always meaningful without context. A good document should be the result of a conversation, not merely the marking of boxes.

In practical terms, a directive that cannot be found at the right time protects no one. The national registry is therefore important. Yet it also requires professional awareness and real-time access. A system in which a person has completed a form but no one checks for it during an emergency admission misses the purpose of the law.

Advance directives also require interpretive humility. No person can be expected to predict every future medical situation. It is therefore useful for the document to reflect not only desired and undesired interventions but also values: what the person considers a meaningful life, what treatment burdens he or she is prepared to bear, and what matters in conditions of uncertainty. Those values can help interpret a situation that was not foreseen.

Advance medical directives are a mechanism of 'future autonomy.' They allow a person to overcome the fact that end-of-life decisions may be required precisely when the ability to speak has been lost. Their strength lies not only in their legal validity but also in the conversation they encourage. Serious completion of the document requires a person to consider scenarios, ask a physician questions, and explain to close relatives what matters most.

The existence of a dedicated registry solves part of the accessibility problem but does not guarantee use. A team must know to check it, the information system must present the information when it is needed, and the person must update details when they change. An excellent document that cannot be found during an emergency admission is almost equivalent to no document at all.

Limited validity recognizes that people change. A position at age fifty may differ from a position at age seventy after an experience of illness. Renewal is not merely a bureaucratic act; it is an opportunity to ask whether the values and the treatments are still understood in the same way. On the other hand, a renewal requirement may weaken the document of a person who did not manage to renew it. Sound policy should therefore include reminders and accessible renewal mechanisms.

One difficulty is that medical scenarios are hard to imagine. A healthy person may say 'I don't want machines' without understanding that two days of ventilation after surgery is very different from permanent ventilation. It is therefore useful to combine specific instructions with statements of values: is the ability to communicate important; what burden is unacceptable; is the person willing to undergo a time-limited trial; how much uncertainty is acceptable? Values help interpret situations that were not expressly listed on the form.

Language is a major barrier. A long medico-legal form can deter even highly educated people. Translation into multiple languages, visual explanations, and a conversation with a family physician can increase use. Accessibility does not reduce seriousness; it allows the document to reflect a choice rather than the person's ability to navigate bureaucracy.

An advance directive should be distinguished from a current medical order. A directive can express a future wish, while a DNR order on a ward is a clinical medical decision in a concrete situation, made in accordance with the law and the patient's wishes. A good system connects the two: when a person arrives with a directive, the team translates it into relevant treatment orders. An on-call nurse in an emergency should not be expected to interpret a long document without a clear order in the medical record.

The family should know that the document exists. Legally, the registry may be sufficient; practically, a conversation with close relatives can prevent surprise. If children first learn of their father's wishes only when clinicians ask them to respect those wishes, resistance may be strong. Advance planning therefore includes family communication as well, to the extent the person wants it.

A directive is not a tool for ending life in a way prohibited by law. It operates within the boundaries established by law. A private document cannot make an unlawful act lawful. This distinction protects clarity: directives are intended to guide treatment decisions, not to create an indirect route to euthanasia.

From the perspective of negligence, two failures are possible: failure to identify an existing document, or unreasonable interpretation of it. The first may be a system or documentation failure; the second may be a professional-legal failure. The best protection is a process: locate the document, verify its validity, assess whether it fits the present situation, document the interpretation, and consult when doubt remains.

Advance directives suit people who want to specify matters in advance. Others prefer to rely on a trusted person who can adapt decisions to future circumstances. For them, a power of attorney may be the more flexible tool. The distinction is not technical; it is a choice between an instruction given in advance and a human representative.

How to Turn a Document Into an Implementable Decision

A good advance medical directive is not a list of slogans. Phrases such as 'I don't want to be a vegetable' or 'don't connect me to machines' express a feeling, but they can be difficult to translate into treatment. A ventilator may provide short-term support that allows full recovery from pneumonia, or it may become prolonged support in irreversible disease. The quality of a directive therefore depends on connecting values to situations and goals: what outcome would be unacceptable to the person, which treatment trials would be acceptable, and what matters most when complete recovery is not possible.

The law gives the document a framework, but medicine interprets it when it encounters reality. Disease does not read the form. A scenario may resemble what the person imagined without being identical, and technology unavailable at the time of signing may create a new option. Periodic updating of directives and discussion with the proxy and family therefore have value. A document renewed after a major change in health status may provide stronger evidence of current wishes.

From a systems perspective, access to the document is part of its practical force. It is not enough for a form to have been signed lawfully if, during an urgent admission, no one knows it exists. A central registry, a marker in the medical record, a copy held by the proxy, and notification of the family physician are layers of safety. Each layer reduces the risk that a decision will be based on assumption rather than documented wishes.

For a lawyer, advance directives create an interpretive question similar to other future-oriented legal documents, but with a decisive difference: the interpretation here affects the person's body in real time. Weight should therefore be given to the language, the circumstances in which the directive was prepared, the explanation the person received, and the continuity of the person's preferences, while avoiding a formalistic reading detached from the medical situation. The goal is not to 'win' a dispute over a clause, but to realize as faithfully as possible the decision the person sought to leave behind.

The two main ways of expressing wishes in advance differ in structure but serve a similar purpose: reducing the need to guess what the person would want once he or she can no longer say so.

Power of Attorney for End-of-Life Decisions

A medical power of attorney under the Dying Patient Law allows a person to choose in advance who will be his or her voice when the person can no longer speak. This is different from a detailed directive. Instead of trying to predict every situation, the person appoints someone trusted to understand the person's values and apply them in future circumstances.

The advantage is flexibility. A proxy can listen to the physicians, understand what has changed, and adapt the decision to reality. The disadvantage is the emotional and interpretive burden. The proxy is not always certain what the person would have wanted, and other family members may disagree. A conversation at the time of appointment is therefore as important as the signature itself.

From a policy perspective, a power of attorney can be simpler and more accessible than a long list of medical instructions. A system that seeks to increase advance planning should therefore offer citizens several routes rather than assume that every person wants or is able to make numerous technical decisions in advance.

The most appropriate representative is not necessarily the closest relative. A spouse may be ideal, but may also be a person who finds the decision unbearable. An adult child may understand the parent's wishes but be in conflict with siblings. It is wise to choose someone able to hear difficult information, ask questions, withstand pressure, and distinguish his or her own wishes from those of the person making the appointment.

A good conversation before the appointment need not be technical. It can focus on goals: would the person accept a small chance of recovery at the price of intensive care; what are his or her views on prolonged dependency; is remaining at home important; what matters religiously? Such information provides the proxy with a compass when reality does not fit a familiar scenario.

A proxy may not demand an unlawful act or medically inappropriate treatment. Authority is limited to decisions the law allows and to the purpose of representation. If the proxy asks for something that contradicts a clear instruction from the person, a problem arises. The team should not immediately take sides, but should review the documents, speak with those involved, and use the appropriate dispute-resolution mechanism if necessary.

A proxy may also change his or her interpretation after hearing the prognosis. This is not necessarily a sign of unreliability. The proxy may previously have failed to understand the difference between temporary and prolonged treatment. The team should therefore provide the proxy with the same type of information it would provide the patient: benefit, burden, alternatives, and what is expected without the treatment. Authority is not a substitute for understanding.

Other family members do not disappear. In practice, their opposition can undermine trust. When possible, it is useful to include them in the explanation while preserving the proxy's legal status. The aim is not to conduct a family vote but to reduce the feeling that a decision was imposed in secret. When the disagreement is deep, a committee can provide a setting in which each side is heard.

Conflicts of interest are also possible. A proxy may be an exhausted primary caregiver or may have a financial interest. The law does not presume dishonesty, but the system must be capable of identifying unusual signs. A request inconsistent with known values, or pressure to end the process rapidly, may justify review. Protecting the person who made the appointment is part of the mechanism.

Documentation matters. The document itself should be accessible, and the medical record should identify the proxy and provide contact information. Searching for a paper at home during a crisis is not a workable system. Digital access, notation in community records, and transfer of information between institutions are operational components that give the document real force.

A power of attorney and advance directives may coexist. If so, their relationship must be understood: is the representative expected to act within specific instructions, and what happens if the representative believes the actual scenario does not fit them? Clear drafting in advance can prevent conflict. The tools should not be viewed as competitors; they can complement one another.

The great strength of a power of attorney is humanity and flexibility; its weakness is interpretation under pressure. For that reason, the law does not leave the representative alone in a difficult dispute. Institutional committees are intended to provide a framework when the wishes, authority, or implementation are unclear.

The Proxy as the Person's Voice, Not as a Substitute for the Person

Appointing a proxy addresses a problem that a written directive cannot solve well: medical reality is too complex for every future scenario to be predicted. A person chosen in advance can hear the physicians, ask questions, and apply the appointing person's values to a new situation. The mechanism's great advantage is flexibility; its greatest risk is that flexibility will become replacement of the person's wishes with the representative's own wishes.

A good choice of proxy is not necessarily the closest relative. The right person should be able to withstand pressure, communicate with the medical team, remember what mattered to the appointing person, and defend a choice that may not match the family's view. Some people prefer a spouse; others choose a sibling, an adult child, or another trusted person. The conversation at the time of appointment is almost as important as the form itself: a proxy who has never heard the person's views may later possess formal authority but no compass.

When both written directives and a proxy exist, their relationship should be examined according to the law and the documents themselves. In general, an explicit document from the patient is direct evidence of wishes, while the proxy assists in implementation and interpretation. If an apparent contradiction arises, it should not immediately be treated as a personal struggle. The document may be old, the circumstances may differ, or the proxy may possess information about a later change of mind that was never documented. A structured inquiry should distinguish a factual claim about later wishes from the representative's personal preference.

The treating team also has a responsibility not to place on the proxy a question that is not truly the proxy's. Instead of asking, 'Do you want us to stop?', it is better to ask, 'What would he tell us if he were able to take part in this conversation?' The change in wording shifts the focus of responsibility and reminds everyone that the subject of the decision is the patient.

Chapter 4

Institutional Committees and the Resolution of Disputes

An institutional committee is an intermediate mechanism between the treatment room and the court. It is close enough to clinical reality to act relatively quickly, yet broad enough to introduce additional perspectives. Its role is not to replace every physician's decision, but to intervene when there is a dispute, uncertainty, or interpretive question that the treating team cannot resolve alone.

A multidisciplinary composition protects against professional blind spots. A physician may focus on survival probabilities, a lawyer on the statute, a social worker on family dynamics, and a nurse on the patient's day-to-day experience. No one holds the entire picture. Yet multidisciplinarity does not guarantee quality if members receive incomplete information or if the culture allows one voice to dominate.

The committee's procedure should be clear. Who may apply, how quickly must it convene, who presents information, is the patient heard, how is the authority of a representative verified, and what is documented? In end-of-life care, time is a substantive element. A decision reached only after the situation has changed is not a good decision. An emergency mechanism is therefore needed for urgent cases alongside a full process when time allows.

Hearing the patient is a basic principle when the patient has capacity. If a committee discusses the patient's rights without allowing participation, it risks becoming a paternalistic mechanism rather than a protective one. When the patient lacks capacity, the sources of the patient's wishes should be presented systematically. 'The family thinks' is not a sufficient category; the committee needs to know which family members, what authority they have, and what evidence supports their account.

Institutional conflict of interest is an inherent risk. The committee operates within a hospital that may itself be a party to the dispute, bear costs, or fear litigation. Transparency, diversity of membership, and the possibility of external review are therefore important to legitimacy. In some cases the mere existence of an external route improves the family's trust even when it is not used.

A committee is not a tribunal for imposing punishment. Its purpose is to resolve rather than accuse. An adversarial approach can harden the position of a family that already fears the system is 'giving up' on a loved one. It is better to begin by asking what each side understands, where the factual accounts differ, and what the actual legal question is. Sometimes the apparent moral disagreement turns out to concern prognosis or the meaning of a treatment.

From a quality perspective, committees should learn from prior cases. Anonymized decisions or summaries of principles can promote consistency among institutions and reduce dependence on who happens to sit on a given day. An internal knowledge base can also identify recurring issues and turn them into training before they reach a crisis.

For a law student, the committee demonstrates administrative-law principles on a clinical scale: authority, fair procedure, evidence, conflicts of interest, reasons, and review. The determination may not always be a judicial judgment, but the same principles of legitimacy apply. A decision without reasons is difficult both to review and to implement.

From a negligence perspective, referral to a committee is not immunity. If the team ignores an urgent condition while waiting for the committee, or provides the committee with incorrect information, responsibility remains. On the other hand, a structured consultation may demonstrate that a serious inquiry was undertaken in a complex case. Again, the quality of the process matters more than checking a box marked 'discussed by committee.'

When the committee finishes its work, the decision must return to the bedside in clear language: what is to be done now, what is not to be done, who is responsible, and when the next reassessment will occur. A legal protocol that is not translated into treatment orders can leave the team in the same confusion. This leads to two complementary chapters: what the law permits a physician to do and what it prohibits.

The Institutional Committee as a Space for Clarification, Not a Small Court

The advantage of an institutional committee is not that it replaces the physician or the patient, but that it creates an organized setting for cases in which ordinary decision-making has become stuck. A dispute may arise from medical uncertainty, differing interpretations of a document, a question of capacity, or conflict among relatives. Each type of dispute requires a different tool, so the committee's first task is to define precisely what is actually contested.

A good process allows every side to be heard without turning the meeting into a hostile arena. The medical facts should be presented in clear language, facts should be separated from estimates, and original documents should be reviewed. When a family representative says 'the physician wants to give up' and the physician says 'the family is demanding futile treatment,' the underlying problem may turn out to be a misunderstanding about the goal of treatment rather than an absolute clash of values.

From the perspective of administrative law and procedural fairness, a committee should be consistent, documented, and free from improper dependence. Its decision should not consist of a vague sentence. It should explain the facts found, the source of authority, and the principal considerations. Giving reasons improves both the quality of the decision and the ability to review it later.

It is equally important to know when a committee is not the solution. An emergency that requires immediate action is not suited to a lengthy process, and a straightforward medical question should not become an ethics proceeding merely because the answer is emotionally difficult to say aloud. A committee is a safety mechanism for borderline situations, not a substitute for the everyday professional responsibility of the team.

Chapter 5

The Limits of the Treating Team's Authority: What Is Permitted, What Is Prohibited, and the Gray Zone

The Scope of Action: Permission, Refusal, Professional Judgment, and Continuation of Care

The options the law gives a physician are not a general 'permission to stop treatment.' They depend on the patient's legal status, the patient's wishes, and the type of intervention. A lawful action therefore begins with identifying the applicable conditions. Teams should avoid shortcuts such as 'the patient is terminal, so we do not resuscitate.' End of life is not an automatic order; it is a framework in which wishes and professional judgment receive weight.

A physician may recommend not starting a treatment that is not expected to achieve a reasonable medical goal. Autonomy does not require the provision of unjustified treatment. The recommendation, however, should be reasoned and should not rest on a value judgment about the person's life. It is better to explain what the treatment can and cannot achieve. The family can then understand that the decision concerns the intervention, not the patient's worth.

Respecting the refusal of a patient with capacity is central. A physician need not 'agree' with the choice in order to respect it, but must ensure understanding, offer alternatives, and continue other care. If a person refuses mechanical ventilation, that does not mean the person refuses oxygen, analgesics, or human presence. Breaking the plan into specific decisions prevents abandonment.

Where the law permits, clinicians may refrain from renewing a cyclical treatment. That distinction requires planning. If a treatment is given in doses or cycles, the point of renewal becomes a decision point. The team should know in advance when that point occurs rather than reach it without having clarified the patient's wishes. Good management makes the law part of the treatment plan rather than a hurried decision at the final moment.

A physician may provide appropriate palliative treatment. There is no need to undertreat pain out of fear that treatment might be viewed as 'bringing death closer' when the treatment is professionally indicated and directed at relief. The physician's duty is to select the dose, monitor, and adjust. Treating suffering is a positive medical action that the law seeks to preserve even when other treatments are limited.

A physician may also propose a time-limited trial of treatment. The law does not require a binary choice in every situation. When uncertainty exists, the parties can agree on goals and duration and then reassess. This is particularly appropriate when the patient is willing to try treatment but does not want prolonged dependency. Documenting the conditions in advance reduces conflict if the trial fails.

Professional freedom includes the right not to perform an act that is medically inappropriate or unlawful. A patient cannot compel a physician in Israel to perform active euthanasia. At the same time, conscientious objection to lawful care requires an institutional response so that rights are not impaired. A physician may not abandon a person merely because the physician disagrees with the person's decision.

Consultation is permitted and often appropriate. Physicians sometimes fear that referral to lawyers or to a committee will appear to show insecurity. The opposite is often true: a complex case justifies review. A second opinion may be part of reasonable care, particularly when the decision is irreversible or when the team and family are in substantial disagreement.

Documentation should avoid vague phrases such as 'supportive care only' when the content is unclear. The record should specify which interventions will be provided, which will not, and what their purposes are. This prevents the night team from having to guess and allows the family to understand the plan. A good record reduces legal risk and clinical error alike.

The scope of lawful action gains meaning only when considered together with its limits. To understand the Israeli compromise, one must know not only what can be done but also what remains outside professional authority even when a patient asks for it. The rest of this chapter therefore places permissions and prohibitions side by side.

Permission, Professional Judgment, and the Duty to Continue Care

When the law permits clinicians to withhold a particular treatment, that does not mean the physician has received 'permission to stop caring.' The decision should be focused on a specific intervention and its purpose. A team can decide not to perform CPR while continuing antibiotics, oxygen, appropriate fluids, pain treatment, and nursing support. It can decide not to initiate new dialysis while still treating breathlessness and anxiety. The distinction between treating the disease and caring for the person becomes especially concrete here.

The law does not replace clinical judgment. If an act is legally permitted but clinically inappropriate, there is no obligation to perform it. By the same token, a physician may not disguise a personal value judgment as a medical determination. The claim that a treatment is 'not appropriate' should relate to the benefit and risk of the intervention, not to age, disability, or an assumption that the person's life is worth less.

Timing matters. A decision made after the patient collapses and the family must answer within minutes is very different from one discussed in advance. One of the most important clinical skills is recognizing the decision point before it becomes a crisis. Recurrent admissions, functional decline, progressive disease, or transition to palliative care are opportunities for conversation. This does not 'bring death forward'; it brings decision-making forward.

From a legal perspective, the strongest protection for a complex decision is consistency between assessment, conversation, and action. If the record says the goal is comfort but invasive procedures continue without explanation, the file contains a contradiction. If CPR is to be withheld but no one tells the team which treatments are to continue, undertreatment becomes a risk. A good document is not merely evidence; it is a tool connecting decision to implementation.

Understanding the scope of action requires seeing both sides at once. Legal or medical permission is incomplete without the boundary on its other side, and a prohibition gains meaning only when it is clear which treatment alternatives remain open.

What a Physician May Not Do

The principal boundary in Israeli law is the prohibition on an act intended to cause the patient's death, even when the patient requests it. Active euthanasia is not permitted, and physician-assisted suicide does not become lawful by virtue of the Dying Patient Law.

The law also restricts discontinuation of continuous treatments where doing so may be regarded as a direct act bringing about death. This is one of the most controversial features of the Israeli arrangement. The structure is intended to preserve a distinction between not prolonging life and an act that actually terminates continuous support.

Another prohibition concerns disregarding the patient's wishes when those wishes are valid and relevant. Protecting life is not a license to impose treatment automatically. When the law recognizes a refusal, treatment contrary to that refusal may infringe autonomy and dignity and may also generate legal responsibility.

Nor may clinicians assume that a wish to die eliminates the need for assessment. When a person expresses despair, pain, anxiety, depression, social distress, and understanding of the condition must be assessed. The law does not allow a shortcut from a verbal wish to an irreversible decision.

These boundaries illustrate the character of the statute: it does not give physicians authority to 'decide who will live.' It creates a framework for respecting wishes concerning treatment while prohibiting the conversion of treatment itself into an intentional means of causing death.

The central prohibition is against an act whose purpose is to cause a person's death. An explicit request, capacity, and suffering do not create an exception in Israel allowing a physician to inject a lethal substance. This boundary distinguishes Israeli law from the Dutch and Belgian models. It should therefore be stated plainly: in some circumstances the law allows life not to be prolonged, but it does not allow killing.

Assistance in suicide likewise receives no authorization under the statute. A physician may not provide a lethal means so that the patient can personally carry out an unlawful act. The distinction between assisted suicide and euthanasia becomes important in comparative law, but in Israel both remain outside the pathway created by the Dying Patient Law.

The law restricts discontinuation of continuous treatments in a way that gives practical effect to the distinction between action and omission. A clinician cannot decide that 'morally there is no difference' and act according to a personal ethical view. As long as the law distinguishes the two, personal ethical judgment is not a substitute for legal compliance. Criticism may lead to reform; it does not authorize violation at the bedside.

It is also prohibited to disregard the valid wishes of a patient merely because the team or family prefers treatment. Invasive treatment without consent can infringe bodily integrity and autonomy. 'Prohibited,' therefore, operates in both directions: it prohibits intentional killing, but it also limits medical power to prolong treatment contrary to the legal framework. The two boundaries together form the compromise.

Loss of capacity does not give the family unlimited authority. The mechanisms of the law must be followed. If a relative asks to stop treatment without a basis in the patient's wishes or legal authority, the team should pause and clarify. Conversely, if the family demands a treatment that is not beneficial, it cannot compel the physician to provide unjustified care.

The law also does not allow basic or palliative care to be discontinued merely because a decision has been made not to prolong life. The duty to treat pain, provide nursing care, and preserve dignity remains. 'No curative treatment' is not a justification for neglect. From the standpoint of professional responsibility, undertreatment of symptoms can constitute a failure even when death is expected.

Sedation may not be used as a cover for an act whose purpose is death. If there is no palliative indication and medication is given in order to cause death, the label does not alter the substance. Sedation protocols, symptom assessment, and dose titration protect the boundary between treatment and killing.

Consent may not be created through misleading information. A family that receives an exaggerated description of hopelessness, or a patient who is not told that an alternative exists, is not making an informed decision. The law examines not only the final act but also the process by which agreement was obtained. In an irreversible field, the reliability of information is both a legal and ethical condition.

A physician may not allow fear of litigation to become the medical objective. Continuing treatment only 'so that no one can say we stopped' may harm the patient. Defensive medicine is not permission to ignore wishes or benefit. The appropriate way to reduce risk is documentation, consultation, and professional decision-making, not unnecessary treatment.

The boundaries described in this chapter lead directly to the statute's most controversial distinction: continuous versus cyclical treatment. The next chapter examines how the legislature attempted to give operational form to the prohibition on direct action and what medical and ethical costs follow from that choice.

The Boundary Between Not Prolonging Life and Causing Death

The prohibitions in Israeli law embody a normative choice: there are acts the system is unwilling to define as part of medical treatment even when the patient requests them. Legally, intention and the type of act matter. There is a difference between deciding not to begin an intervention intended to postpone death and taking an act whose direct purpose is to cause death. The distinction is not always philosophically simple, but the statute uses it as a practical boundary.

The difficulty is especially evident when treatment has already begun. When a machine or medication continuously supports a vital function, stopping it may bring death rapidly. Israeli law sought to address this difficulty through distinctive classifications of treatment and through the idea of cyclical treatment. The distinction can be criticized, but physicians do not have freedom to disregard it merely because they prefer another ethical model.

A legal prohibition does not preclude aggressive treatment of symptoms. A common error is to fear that any substantial dose of analgesia in a dying patient is 'too close' to euthanasia. Professional palliative treatment is based on therapeutic purpose, appropriate dosing, and monitoring. When the intention is to relieve suffering and the treatment meets professional standards, it should be distinguished from an act intended to cause death.

For lawyers, this is an area in which factual description determines classification. The phrase 'they disconnected him' is insufficient: what was disconnected, at what stage, under what decision, what was the purpose of the act, and what did the law provide concerning that type of treatment? Only after those facts are separated can responsibility be analyzed. Emotionally loaded public language is not a substitute for precise facts.

Chapter 6

Continuous and Cyclical Treatment and Types of Life-Prolonging Care: The Israeli Distinction Tested in Clinical Practice

One of the distinctions most closely associated with Israeli law is that between continuous and cyclical treatment. Cyclical treatment is administered at intervals at which a decision can be made whether to renew it; continuous treatment operates without interruption, and stopping it is a distinct act. The distinction was designed to create room for deciding not to renew treatment without treating every case as a direct act of ending life.

The practical result can be complex. The distinction may create an incentive to think in advance about the structure of treatment and to plan pauses or cycles. It also requires teams to understand the legal classification rather than rely on intuition. An error in classification may result either in prolonged treatment contrary to the patient's wishes or in discontinuation that does not conform to law.

The issue is not merely technical. It concerns whether morality should treat 'doing' and 'not doing' differently. The normative chapter will examine that question in depth; here it is enough to understand that the Israeli legislature gave the distinction practical legal force.

A conventional ventilator is an example of continuous treatment. Once the patient depends on it, turning off the machine is a clear act. Dialysis or medication given in doses may be viewed as cyclical. Yet medicine does not always fit neat categories. Continuous treatment can include adjustments, and a cyclical treatment may be so essential that death follows quickly without it. Classification therefore requires understanding both the technology and the law.

Supporters of the distinction attribute significance to the active act itself. For them, turning off life support that immediately results in death is experienced differently from not administering the next dose. The distinction may be grounded in Jewish law, moral intuition, or institutional concern about blurring the line toward killing. A legal system may give weight to that intuition even if philosophers disagree with it.

Technological solutions, such as timers, attempt to alter the structure of the act without changing the purpose of treatment. If a device operates in cycles that require renewal, a legal decision can be made not to renew. But such a solution raises questions: does it truly change the moral character of the decision or merely its description; is it safe; and who bears responsibility at the point of renewal? Technology becomes a legal instrument as well as a medical one.

In ward practice, the distinction requires advance planning and documentation. It is not enough to write 'do not renew' without identifying when, which treatment, and under what conditions. A new shift needs to know what is considered a cycle and what was decided. An error can be irreversible in either direction.

The distinction also affects the conversation with the patient before treatment begins. If the possibilities for stopping treatment later are limited, that information should be explained. Consent to start treatment without information about limitations on stopping it is incomplete. This is especially relevant to a treatment trial intended to be temporary. The person needs to understand not only the chance of success but also the options if the trial fails.

From a negligence perspective, classification can become relevant when treatment continues contrary to the patient's wishes because the team failed to plan correctly, or when treatment is discontinued in a manner that does not comply with law. Medico-legal expertise requires understanding the technology rather than relying on labels. A lawyer may need to read device instructions, treatment records, and time points.

The continuous-versus-cyclical distinction also illustrates a broader question: should law embed a moral distinction by means of technology? If future medicine introduces automated devices or new forms of support, statutory definitions may become outdated. Periodic review is therefore essential to ensure that the law continues to achieve its purpose rather than merely preserve categories created in 2005.

Once the classification is understood, the analysis must move from the category to the treatments themselves. Each intervention - ventilation, resuscitation, dialysis, antibiotics, chemotherapy, fluids, and nutrition - carries different goals and burdens, so serious legal analysis must descend from the general concept to the bedside.

The Israeli Distinction Tested by Technology

The distinction between continuous and cyclical treatment arose as an attempt to reconcile different moral positions. In practice it seeks to create a situation in which unwanted treatment can end at a natural point of renewal without a direct act stopping an uninterrupted flow. Medical technology, however, does not always fit comfortably into such categories: pumps, ventilators, continuous dialysis, and timed treatments blur the lines.

The advantage of the distinction is that it provides clinicians and society with a relatively clear rule of action in sensitive situations. Its disadvantage is that it may attach major moral significance to a technical feature of a device. If two treatments achieve the same goal but one operates continuously and the other in cycles, it is reasonable to ask whether the legal result should differ. This is one area in which the gap between statutory language and technological development may widen over time.

The solution is not free interpretation by each ward. As long as the law remains in force, changes should occur through authorized guidelines, legal interpretation, or legislative amendment. Otherwise, clinically similar patients could receive different decisions depending on the institution or the technical creativity of the team. In an irreversible field, a high degree of consistency is especially important.

A future Israeli debate should ask whether to preserve the distinction, update its definitions, or move toward a test based more directly on treatment purpose, the patient's wishes, and causal relationship. Every alternative has a price: a simple technical rule may be artificial, while a flexible value-based test may be less predictable. This is a good example of why medical legislation must change cautiously together with the technology it regulates.

Artificial Ventilation, Resuscitation, Dialysis, Antibiotics, Chemotherapy, Fluids, and Nutrition: Analysis by Treatment Type

End-of-life decisions do not occur only at the level of the abstract term 'treatment.' Each intervention has a different meaning. Ventilation may be a bridge to recovery from a reversible infection or prolonged support in irreversible disease. Dialysis may permit independent life or impose a heavy burden during the dying process. Chemotherapy may cure, prolong life, or impose burden without benefit, depending on the disease and its stage.

Resuscitation is one of the interventions that requires advance planning. A DNR decision concerns a specific action in the event of cardiac or respiratory arrest; it is not an instruction to stop other care. Confusing DNR with 'do not treat' is both a professional and a communication failure.

Antibiotics illustrate the importance of treatment purpose. In a dying patient they may prolong the process without improvement, but sometimes they relieve symptoms caused by infection. The decision is therefore not ideological. The appropriate questions are what goal the treatment is expected to achieve and what the person prefers.

Fluids and nutrition are particularly sensitive. A family may experience their discontinuation as starvation or dehydration, even though during some stages of dying the body no longer processes food and fluids in the usual way and excess administration can cause edema, secretions, and discomfort. Conversely, this should not be turned into a blanket rule. Each case requires clinical assessment.

Prolonged ventilation also raises questions of weaning, tracheostomy, and transfer to a chronic-care setting. A decision to initiate ventilation in a borderline situation should therefore include, at the outset, a conversation about the purpose of the trial and what will happen if that purpose is not achieved. 'We'll try and see' without defining what counts as success can become an intervention with no agreed way out.

The common principle is that the treatment's name does not decide the outcome. Medical condition, benefit, burden, wishes, and legal status must be considered together. That is the essence of individualized end-of-life medicine.

With mechanical ventilation, invasive and non-invasive ventilation and short- and long-term support should be distinguished. A patient with reversible pneumonia is not in the same position as a person with advanced neurodegenerative disease. The conversation should include not only the chance of surviving the hospitalization but also the chance of coming off the ventilator and returning to a functional level. For some people survival with a tracheostomy is acceptable; for others it is an outcome they do not want.

Resuscitation requires a clear order. DNR refers to an event of cardiac or respiratory arrest and does not mean 'do not treat.' A person with a DNR order may receive antibiotics, dialysis, surgery, or intensive care if those treatments are consistent with the person's goals. Confusing the order with a global limitation of care can lead to neglect. Decisions about other treatments should therefore be documented separately.

Dialysis presents a repeated burden. Treatment can prolong life for a long period, but in advanced illness it may cause weakness, hypotension, and frequent travel. When a decision is made not to start or renew dialysis, symptom management for renal failure must be planned. Discontinuing a treatment is not discontinuing medicine.

Antibiotics are sometimes regarded as simple treatment and therefore given automatically. At the end of life, however, their purpose should be explicit: are clinicians trying to cure an infection to prolong life, or to relieve a symptom? Sometimes an untreated infection may permit a relatively natural death without aggressive intervention; sometimes a short course improves comfort. There is no single rule for every infection.

Chemotherapy and other oncological treatments require distinguishing lines of treatment intended for cure, life prolongation, and symptom relief. When the chance of response is small and toxicity is high, presenting 'another treatment' as a neutral option can postpone an important conversation. The oncologist should explain the expected gain in time and its price, not merely state that another drug is available.

Intravenous fluids at the end of life evoke an image of preventing thirst, but the sensation of thirst is not always improved by fluid loading. Oral care, moisture, and ice can be meaningful, while excess fluids may worsen edema and secretions. The decision should be clinical rather than symbolic. Families should be told that not providing an IV infusion is not necessarily 'dehydrating' the patient.

Artificial nutrition is even more sensitive because food is associated with love and care. Tube feeding can save life when swallowing is temporarily impaired, but in some end-of-life states benefit is limited and risks remain. Hand feeding according to ability and comfort should be distinguished from medical nutrition through a tube, and the specific legal framework should be examined. Language that respects the symbolic meaning of food can reduce conflict.

Chronic preventive medications are an often-forgotten category. Statins, vitamins, long-term preventive medications, or routine tests may lose relevance when life expectancy is short. Deprescribing is part of quality care: reducing medication burden that no longer contributes to the treatment goal. This is different from discontinuing a medication that relieves symptoms or prevents immediate suffering.

Blood transfusions, pacemakers, and implanted devices also require planning. An implantable defibrillator can deliver painful shocks in the final hours if it has not been adjusted to the goals of care. Turning off the shock function is not necessarily the same as discontinuing pacing. The team should understand the device and involve a specialist. Technology that is not reviewed can contradict the entire comfort plan.

The Benefit-Burden Profile of Each Intervention

Assessment of treatment at the end of life requires more than asking whether it 'prolongs life.' Clinicians must consider the probability that the treatment will achieve a goal that matters to the patient, the expected duration of the benefit, and the cost or burden. CPR can restore circulation without necessarily restoring consciousness or independence; ventilation can bridge a temporary failure but can also lead to weeks in intensive care; dialysis can relieve symptoms of renal failure but require repeated transport and treatments. Describing only the biological outcome is not sufficient for informed consent.

A practical test can be built around four recurring questions: what goal is the intervention intended to achieve; what is the probability and expected time to achieve it; what burden does it impose; and what will count as a stopping point if the goal is not achieved? This structure allows clinicians and patients to discuss each treatment individually without turning the choice into an all-or-nothing package.

Brief Case: A Time-Limited Trial of Treatment

A patient with respiratory failure agrees to a short trial of intensive treatment to determine whether reversible recovery is possible. The clinical goals, duration of the trial, and criteria for failure are defined in advance. The case illustrates why a decision to start treatment should not be detached from the question of how it will later be evaluated, and how the Israeli distinction between continuous and cyclical treatment can affect the decision from the moment the treatment is first offered.

The unifying principle is not a list of what is 'permitted' or 'prohibited' according to the name of a treatment. The questions are what the goal is, what the benefit is, what burden is imposed, what the person wants, and how the intervention is legally classified. Once each treatment is analyzed in this way, disputes can be addressed more effectively. The next chapter turns to treatment of suffering - particularly pain, morphine, and sedation - where legal anxiety itself can lead to undertreatment.

Chapter 7

Pain, Morphine, and Palliative Sedation

Pain is one of the greatest fears people face in terminal illness, and at times it is also a source of requests to die. Proper pain treatment is therefore both a medical duty and a condition for an honest discussion of wishes. A person who is not receiving basic relief from suffering is not choosing from the same position as a person who has had access to optimal palliative care.

Opioids such as morphine sometimes carry a stigma among families: 'Once they give morphine, it is the end.' This belief can lead to undertreatment. The professional goal is to tailor the dose to relieve pain or breathlessness, with monitoring and planning. The fact that the drug is potent does not turn the treatment into killing.

Palliative sedation requires a different threshold because it can reduce wakefulness and communication. The team should establish that the symptom is refractory, define the therapeutic goal, and ensure that the patient or representative understands the implications. The process should be documented especially carefully when deep and continuous sedation is considered.

From a legal perspective, professional intent and conformity with the standard of care are central. Giving a dose for the purpose of relief differs from giving a dose for the purpose of causing death. Documentation of the indication, assessment, dose, and response is therefore not merely a clinical tool but also evidence of the nature of the act.

The discussion of pain is a reminder that law cannot consist only of prohibitions. If a system prohibits assistance in dying but fails to provide adequate treatment for suffering, it does not fully protect human dignity. Protection of life must also include the quality of care during the life that remains.

Morphine is a public symbol of the end of life and often a source of fear. Families worry that it 'stops breathing,' and clinicians sometimes fear that it will appear as though they hastened death. Professional care should dismantle the fear: morphine is used for pain and dyspnea, the dose is individualized, and the decision is symptom-based. Arbitrary dosing is unacceptable, but leaving a person to suffer because of a myth is also unacceptable.

Pain assessment is difficult when the person cannot speak. Clinicians rely on behavior, facial expression, movement, vocalization, and other signs, but no tool is perfect. In a person with dementia or reduced consciousness, knowledge of the person's usual behavior and input from the family are important. Undertreatment is common when inability to communicate is mistaken for absence of pain.

Breathlessness is an especially frightening symptom. Oxygen is not always the only answer, and in some situations appropriately dosed opioids can reduce the sensation of dyspnea. Positioning, airflow, the environment, and calm support also matter. When the goal is comfort, oxygen saturation is not the only outcome; the person's experience matters.

Titration is what distinguishes professional treatment from uncontrolled use. Dosing begins according to the clinical situation, response is assessed, and the dose or drug is adjusted as needed. Kidney and liver function, age, and prior opioid exposure all matter. Documenting the indication and dose is particularly important at the end of life because death may occur close to administration and later raise questions.

Palliative sedation enters the picture when a severe symptom remains refractory. It is not a mandatory stage for every patient and is not a solution for staff convenience. The decision should address the goal of treatment, alternatives, desired depth, and consent whenever possible. In the final hours of life, the process may be adapted to urgency without abandoning its principles.

Pain management is not the physician's task alone. Nurses identify change, administer treatment under orders, assess response, and report what they see. If orders are too rigid, a patient may wait hours between doses. A good palliative plan therefore includes appropriate ranges and clear instructions that fit the legal and professional framework.

A family may ask that the team 'not give too much' so the person can remain awake. The team should determine what the patient wants. Sometimes a balance can be found between alertness and relief; sometimes the severity of pain requires deeper treatment. When the patient has capacity, the decision is not the family's, but explanation is important so that guilt does not develop.

Under the law, pain treatment does not become prohibited merely because there is a theoretical risk of respiratory effect. Purpose and professional standard are critical. Good intentions alone are not enough; the dose must also be reasonable. Medical responsibility is assessed through the process, not simply by the fact that a terminally ill patient died after treatment.

Undertreatment can itself be harm. Severe pain that could have been relieved is not an unavoidable fate. A system that responds to legal anxiety by routinely using doses that are too low harms patients. Training, protocols, and access to palliative consultation reduce risk and increase clinicians' confidence.

The most important principle is that sedation is not a shortcut when a difficult conversation, staff shortage, or family distress makes care more complicated. It is a clinical intervention for a patient suffering from a refractory symptom. Precisely because it can remove the outward expression of suffering, it requires caution: the team must make sure it is not sedating a problem that could reasonably be addressed in another way. When the criteria are met, however, refusing sedation out of legal fear can leave a person in avoidable suffering, and that too is a morally and professionally significant decision.

High-quality documentation should allow an outside reviewer to reconstruct the decision: what the symptom was, why it was considered refractory, what alternatives were tried or considered, who participated in the discussion, what the patient's wishes were, what depth of sedation was planned, and how the response was assessed. Such documentation protects both the patient and the team. It prevents accepted treatment of suffering from later appearing to be an unexplained act performed close to death.

Consent is central when the person still has capacity. As far as the clinical situation permits, the patient should understand the purpose of sedation, how much it is expected to reduce wakefulness, whether it is temporary or may become continuous, and what alternatives exist. When the patient lacks capacity, prior wishes and the authority of the representative must be examined within the legal framework. Even then, 'the family asked us to sedate' is not enough. The treating team must identify a medical indication and state a clear therapeutic purpose.

Decisions about artificial fluids and nutrition should not automatically be absorbed into the decision about sedation. A person may require deep sedation while fluids are beneficial, non-beneficial, or burdensome depending on the clinical condition. Contemporary European palliative guidance emphasizes that this question requires separate consideration. This avoids a common mistake: treating sedation as a package from which discontinuation of every other treatment automatically follows. Each intervention should be assessed according to its purpose, expected benefit, and burden.

One of the important distinctions from euthanasia lies in the structure of the decision. In sedation, the direct goal is to reduce the experience of suffering; death is not the means used to achieve that goal. Drug selection, dose escalation, and monitoring should therefore be explained in terms of response to the symptom. If the dose is chosen by asking, 'How much is needed to make the patient die?', the act is no longer palliative treatment. If it is chosen by asking, 'How much is needed to relieve the suffering?', it belongs to a different professional framework of intent, standard, and documentation.

Proportionality means that the depth and duration of sedation should match the degree of suffering and the therapeutic objective. If relief can be achieved at a level that allows some communication, there is no automatic justification for deeper suppression of consciousness. Conversely, when dyspnea, delirium, pain, or another severe symptom remains uncontrolled despite appropriate care, deep sedation may be justified. The goal is not to reach a predetermined level of consciousness but to use the lowest intensity that provides adequate relief.

The updated framework of the European Association for Palliative Care emphasizes two principles that help define the boundary: refractoriness and proportionality. A 'refractory symptom' is not merely a severe symptom. It is suffering that cannot be adequately relieved within a reasonable time by accepted measures without imposing an unacceptable burden. Before deep sedation, the team should therefore ask what treatments have been tried, what options remain, whether further consultation is available, and what the patient personally regards as intolerable.

Public discussion often treats palliative sedation as a single act, but clinically there are different depths and durations. Sometimes it means a mild, temporary reduction in alertness to control an acute symptom; in other situations, deep continuous sedation until death is required. The deeper and more prolonged the intervention, the greater the importance of an orderly decision-making process, because the cost is not only a drug effect but the possible loss of communication, leave-taking, eating, and the ability to actively revise a decision.

Deep Continuous Sedation: When Relief of Suffering Requires Surrendering Wakefulness

From a Nursing Perspective: Symptom Management Around the Clock

A good palliative decision is tested not only by the wording of the order but by the ability to carry it out around the clock. An order for 'morphine as needed' is insufficient if there is no clinical definition of need, dose range, interval, route of administration, and instruction for when to contact a physician. When the patient cannot report symptoms verbally, nurses rely on breathing pattern, facial expression, restlessness, guarding, changes in pulse, and knowledge of the patient's baseline behavior.

In a dying patient, restlessness is not always pain. It can result from delirium, urinary retention, constipation, hypoxia, fever, drug withdrawal, an uncomfortable position, or anxiety. Giving an opioid for every episode of agitation may be incorrect treatment; on the other hand, withholding it because of an unfounded fear of hastening death can leave pain and breathlessness untreated. Good nursing assessment connects signs, history, treatment response, and family reports.

Route of administration also matters. When swallowing is unsafe, a plan built around oral medication may fail precisely when it is most needed. The route should be adapted to the patient's condition and care setting, and both staff and family should know what may be given and when. In home care, family teaching is a safety component: it reduces fear of medication, helps prevent double dosing, and clarifies whom to call when symptoms are not controlled.

The nursing record has special legal significance here. When death occurs shortly after medication, documentation of the symptom before the dose, the amount given, route, subsequent assessment, and physician's order helps reconstruct the purpose and reasonableness of the act. The record is not written merely 'for defense'; it is written to ensure continuity of care. Its value as strong retrospective evidence follows from professional practice.

This preserves the division of labor among the book's chapters. The conceptual discussion of sedation addresses intent, proportionality, and double effect; here the emphasis is on what clinicians actually do to make relief of suffering safe, continuous, and controlled.

Brief Case: Sedation Intended to Relieve Suffering

A dying patient has severe dyspnea that does not respond to ordinary measures. After palliative assessment, a graded sedation plan is established to relieve suffering, with documentation of the symptom, alternatives, consent, and response to treatment. The case illustrates that the distinction between sedation and killing does not depend on the name of the drug alone, but on indication, intent, dose, titration, and monitoring.

Pain and sedation show why law must leave room for medicine. If every dosing decision required legal approval, care would suffer. The law should define boundaries, and the profession should fill the space within them through standards of care. The next chapter moves from the physician-patient relationship to another center of power: the family.

Chapter 8

The Role of the Family and What Happens When the Family and the Patient Want Different Things

Families are deeply involved in medical care in Israel. That involvement can be a major source of support, but also of tension. Sometimes relatives ask the physician, 'Don't tell him he is sick,' in an effort to protect the patient even though the patient has a right to information. Sometimes the patient asks not to be ventilated while family members demand that the team 'do everything.' And sometimes the situation is reversed: the patient wants treatment while an exhausted family prefers limits.

The basic principle is that a patient with capacity is the decision-maker. The family's love does not replace the patient. The team should listen to relatives and give space to their difficulty, but should not transfer to them authority they do not possess. When the patient lacks capacity, the family's role depends on the legal mechanisms and on evidence of the patient's wishes.

It is important to distinguish a value conflict from a misunderstanding. A family demanding resuscitation may believe that the physician is proposing 'not to save' the patient, when the clinical assessment is actually that CPR will not restore meaningful function and will cause trauma. Clear information can sometimes transform conflict into agreement.

Guilt is often present. A relative may fear that agreeing not to continue treatment means 'killing' the patient. The team's role is to clarify who is making which decision and what the disease process itself is doing. The family should not be burdened with a moral responsibility that is not truly theirs.

When disagreement persists, additional professionals should be involved: a senior physician, palliative care, social work, ethics support, or an institutional committee. The goal is not to defeat the family but to reach a decision that respects the patient and is professionally and legally grounded.

Family is often the patient's most important source of support, but the end of life can expose deep differences. One child wants treatment to continue, another wants comfort care, and the spouse knows that the patient did not want prolonged intervention. There is no need to view disagreement as family failure; it is a human response to fear and anticipatory grief. The team's task is to organize the discussion around the patient's wishes and the medical facts.

When the patient has capacity, authority is straightforward: the patient's wishes are central. Yet a person may want the family to share in decision-making. That preference should be respected. Autonomy does not require individualism. The distinction is that family involvement arises from the patient's choice, not from an assumption that the family always decides.

When the patient lacks capacity, relatives may serve as sources of information or as representatives according to their legal status. These functions should be kept separate. A person may know very well what a parent wanted without being the appointed proxy; a proxy may have legal authority but need information from siblings. A sound process gathers knowledge while preserving formal authority.

The phrase 'do everything' needs to be unpacked. Sometimes the family means 'do not abandon him,' not 'perform CPR under all circumstances.' If the team explains what will continue - pain control, oxygen, nursing care, presence - agreement may become possible without arguing over a slogan. Likewise, a request to 'stop everything' may mean 'stop the suffering,' not stop food, touch, or comfort medications.

Guilt can shape decisions. A child who has not been present during recent months may demand aggressive treatment in order to feel that something was done; an exhausted primary caregiver may long for the ordeal to end quickly. These reactions should not be judged, but the team should recognize that emotion is not necessarily the patient's wish. Individual conversations with family members may help.

Family conflict can become clinical when different staff members identify with different relatives. A nurse who knows the patient well may support limiting treatment, while an on-call physician may prefer continuation until a formal decision is made. A team meeting before a large family discussion helps prevent the family from receiving contradictory messages.

Family structure also matters. Unmarried partners, blended families, estranged relationships, or a close friend may have significance that is not reflected in biological kinship. The law determines authority, but medicine should understand the patient's network of relationships. The person the patient trusted in life may be an important source of information even if not a 'first-degree relative.'

When exploitation is suspected, the team has a duty to protect. Financial pressure, violence, or controlling behavior are not merely private matters if they influence medical decisions. Social work, an institutional committee, and legal consultation may be needed. Protecting vulnerable people is part of autonomy, because a choice made under coercion is not truly a choice.

Families also need to know what to expect after a decision is made. If treatment will not be renewed, relatives should understand how symptoms will be managed and what signs of dying may occur. Lack of preparation can lead to a demand to return to aggressive treatment at a moment of fear even when the earlier decision was agreed upon. Continuing support matters as much as the initial discussion.

Managing Family Conflict Without Losing the Patient

A family is not a single body. Spouses, children, and siblings may hold different memories of the patient's wishes and carry different burdens. One person who lived with the patient may know years of ordinary conversations; another arrives from far away and suddenly encounters the severity of the illness. Such differences can quickly become accusations about love, guilt, or interests. A professional team should recognize the complexity without becoming a judge of the family's relationships.

An effective family meeting begins with shared facts: what the illness is, what has changed, and what the realistic options are. The discussion then turns to what is known about the patient's values and wishes. Only after that should the recommendation be presented. The order matters, because if the family is asked to 'decide' before it understands the clinical picture, relatives may be left with the feeling that they caused the death of someone they love.

When a relative demands treatment that the team regards as non-beneficial, the team should ask what lies behind the request. The person may need time to say goodbye; may fear that limiting treatment will cause suffering; or may not understand that the intervention cannot restore the patient to the prior state. Addressing the emotional question can resolve what initially appears to be a legal dispute.

If disagreement remains, the discussion should return to the framework of authority. Who may represent the patient? What do existing documents establish? What are the limits of professional clinical judgment? It is not the family's role to demand a prohibited act, and it is not the team's role to erase the family's voice because that voice is difficult. A respectful process protects both the patient's rights and the family's ability to leave the experience feeling that it was heard.

After death, the quality of the process affects bereavement. A family that felt informed and believed it helped respect the patient may cope differently from a family that feels the decision was imposed. There is no guarantee that guilt will disappear, but transparency and presence can reduce trauma. The team's work is therefore not merely to execute orders; it is to accompany people through the process.

The next chapter explains how responsibility for that accompaniment is divided among the different professions.

Chapter 9

The Roles of Physicians, Nurses, Social Workers, and Palliative Care Teams

End-of-life care is a multidisciplinary field. The physician is responsible for diagnosis, prognosis, and major medical decisions, but is not the only professional who sees the patient. Nurses are often at the bedside for long periods, identify suffering, hear things the patient does not say during a physician's visit, and mediate between family and team. Social workers bring information about relationships, support, anxiety, and burden. Palliative care teams integrate symptoms, goals, and communication.

The nurse's unique contribution is not only the amount of time spent at the bedside but the continuity of information. Nurses can detect a gap between a general order and the patient's response, between a decision formulated during a daytime meeting and the reality of the night shift, and between a family's report and a functional change observed directly. When such information is communicated and documented in time, it can alter both the clinical assessment and the quality of the legal decision-making process.

Nurses sometimes experience moral distress when they feel that the treatment they are asked to provide is prolonging suffering or, conversely, that limitations are being imposed too quickly. A high-quality system should allow them to voice a professional view rather than treating them as mere executors. Clear decisions and documentation reduce the gap between those who decide and those who carry out the plan.

Physicians need a skill that is not always taught enough: talking about prognosis. A phrase such as 'there is nothing more to do' is not only inaccurate but harmful. It is better to explain what is no longer beneficial and what will still be done. Communication is part of treatment, not a soft addition to it.

Social workers and psychologists may identify family pressure, financial fear, loneliness, or a sense of being a burden. This information is especially important when a patient asks to stop treatment. The question 'Is this a free choice?' sometimes requires understanding the surrounding environment, not merely testing cognitive capacity.

Palliative care teams help translate a general goal into a concrete plan: what treatment continues, what is stopped, how pain is managed, who is available at home, and what to do in a crisis. In this way, a legal decision becomes a clinical course that does not abandon the patient.

More broadly, the quality of end-of-life care depends less on one professional hero and more on team culture. Law can define boundaries, but the way a person experiences the final days depends on the people who implement those boundaries.

Transfer of Responsibility Between Shifts and Care Settings

One of the greatest risks at the end of life is not a wrong decision but a correct decision that is lost in transit. A patient may move from a ward to intensive care, from hospital to community care, or from the day team to the night team. At every transition there is a risk that the treatment goal will be reduced to an ambiguous line in the chart. Decisions about limits of treatment should therefore be transmitted as a structured clinical message: the patient's condition, the patient's wishes, which treatments fit the goal, what has been decided not to do, and who should be contacted if circumstances change.

A good handoff is not satisfied with a code such as 'supportive care' or 'do not resuscitate.' The next team needs to know the rationale and what remains active: pain treatment, antibiotics in defined circumstances, fluids as appropriate, oxygen, palliative review, or a goal of remaining at home. Such detail prevents two opposite errors - automatic escalation that contradicts the person's wishes, and excessive reduction in care because someone interpreted a limit on one intervention as abandonment of treatment altogether.

Nurses have a central safety role because they see the distance between the written plan and what actually happens. A change in consciousness, uncontrolled pain, a family member who produces a new document, or an on-call physician unfamiliar with the decision are situations in which a clear escalation mechanism is needed. Continuity of care is not merely administrative; it is how an ethical and legal decision is preserved throughout the day and night.

Cross-Checking and Preventing Information Failures

From a risk-management perspective, a multidisciplinary team also creates mutual checking. A physician can misunderstand the patient's values; a nurse may not know the prognosis; a relative may forget a signed document. A brief, documented team discussion at a major decision point can reveal a gap before it becomes harm. This is the proper use of a system: not to diffuse responsibility, but to connect information so responsibility can be exercised more effectively.

The legal section therefore ends not with a statutory provision but with the team. Law operates through people. The next chapter asks whether the legal mechanism actually reaches the public and the wards: how many people know about it, why relatively few plan in advance, where gaps arise, and what happens when legal anxiety or organizational culture overrides a right that exists on paper.

Chapter 10

Awareness and Advance Planning for the End of Life

How Many Israelis Actually Know the Law?

A law can create a detailed right and still remain almost invisible to the people meant to use it. One of the central problems in advance care planning is the awareness gap: many people discover advance medical directives and powers of attorney only after serious illness has already developed, and sometimes only when the person finds it difficult to address the issue or has already lost capacity.

A 2025 document of the Knesset Research and Information Center, written roughly twenty years after enactment of the law, examined its implementation and the use of advance-directive mechanisms. The very need for renewed review shows that the challenge has moved from asking whether advance planning should be permitted to asking how to turn it into a tool that people actually use.

Lack of awareness is not caused only by poor public information. People tend to postpone conversations about death. Even a person who prepares a financial will may never think about a future loss of medical decision-making capacity. In the health system, a short family-physician visit usually focuses on the immediate problem rather than on end-of-life planning. This creates a paradox: when a person is well and able to decide calmly, the subject is not raised; once the person is ill, time is short and the emotional burden is greater.

Awareness should not be built through fear. A more effective approach is to present advance directives as part of responsible health planning, similar to choosing a proxy or planning chronic care. A person does not have to believe death is imminent in order to decide who should speak if consciousness or capacity is lost.

Language also matters. The expression 'dying patient' can distance a healthy person even though the document is meant to be completed before that status exists. Public information should separate the time of signing from the time of activation: the directive is not a declaration that the person has given up on life; it is a future instruction that takes effect only under defined conditions.

A system that wants to increase use should turn the conversation from a passive right into an active service: provide reminders, explain the options, make completion accessible, and ensure that the document can be found later. Otherwise autonomy remains mainly on paper.

The gap between the existence of a law and public familiarity with it is a problem of effective rights. A person cannot use advance directives if never told they exist, especially if first exposed to them during a crisis. The 2025 Knesset Research and Information Center document examined implementation and emphasized the need to look not only at the legal arrangement but also at the extent of actual use. Such measurement asks whether the law has reached citizens or remains primarily in the hands of experts.

Awareness is not binary. A person may know that there is an 'end-of-life form' but not understand when it applies, or may mistakenly think it permits euthanasia. A survey that measures only whether people have heard of the law can therefore overstate familiarity. Good public information should test understanding: who may complete the documents, what is the difference between a directive and a power of attorney, when does the document become operative, and what does it not permit.

Family physicians are well placed to raise the subject before serious illness, but short appointments and urgent priorities make this difficult. Other contact points are possible: periodic examinations at a certain age, repeated hospitalizations, diagnosis of an advanced chronic disease, or admission to a residential-care setting. The goal is not to frighten people, but to make medical planning a normal part of life management.

Hospitals can offer information at admission, but the timing is sensitive. A patient arriving for surgery may interpret an end-of-life form as a suggestion that the team expects death. It is therefore important to distinguish general information from a personal clinical conversation. An accessible information sheet or referral to an official website may be appropriate, while a discussion of treatment goals requires context.

Awareness differs between population groups. Language, health literacy, trust in the health system, and digital access all matter. If information exists only in legal Hebrew on a website, it will not reach the whole public. Equitable policy requires translation, plain-language materials, and channels that are not digital only.

Professionals also do not always master the details. A physician may know the law in general but not know how to access the registry or how long a document remains valid. One-time training is insufficient in a field that does not arise every day. Electronic reminders, short protocols, and access to consultation can turn theoretical knowledge into practice.

Public communication should avoid political framing. If a campaign is presented as 'how not to prolong life,' some members of the public may fear that the state is trying to save treatment costs. A better framing is that the process records a person's wishes, whether the person wants to avoid certain interventions or wants to make clear that they should be provided. The law does not belong to only one side of the public debate.

The success of public education can be measured not only by the number of forms completed but by their quality and accessibility. A form signed without understanding is not an achievement. It is worth asking whether people spoke with their families, whether documents are actually in the registry, and whether clinicians can retrieve them when needed. These measures bring evaluation closer to the law's real purpose.

From a legal perspective, low public awareness does not invalidate the statute, but it may expose a policy failure. When the state creates a complex right that depends on prior action by the citizen, it is reasonable to expect investment in accessibility. Otherwise people who know physicians and lawyers benefit more than those who are less connected to the system.

The awareness gap leads to the next question: even people who know about the option sometimes postpone planning. The reason is not only bureaucracy. Death is a subject people avoid, and medicine needs to understand the psychology of that avoidance in order to design a process people can actually use.

Measuring Awareness Rather Than Relying on Public Impression

When we say that the public 'does not know the law,' it is important to define what knowledge means. A person may know that it is possible to leave instructions in advance but not know the conditions; may know the phrase 'living will' but not know where a document is deposited; or may mistakenly believe the law permits euthanasia. Real research on awareness should therefore distinguish name recognition, understanding of content, and the practical ability to use the right.

Implementation data matter because they allow the gap between a formal right and an effective right to be measured. The number of deposited forms, the characteristics of users, renewal rates, and the ability of clinicians to retrieve the document in time are different indicators. Even low use does not necessarily prove failure: some people do not wish to plan in advance. The relevant question is whether those who do wish to plan can do so without unnecessary barriers.

Awareness is influenced by how the state presents the service. If information appears only on a dedicated website that citizens must search for themselves, nearly all responsibility is shifted to the individual. By contrast, incorporating explanation into medical encounters, health-plan services, or the process surrounding a major diagnosis makes the right more accessible. The difference is not merely promotional; it concerns equality in the practical exercise of rights.

Evaluation of the law should therefore ask not only how many people signed, but who never reached the information and why. Language barriers, digital literacy, age, accessibility, and cultural discomfort may all explain low use. Good policy does not force a person to decide in advance about dying; it ensures that choosing not to sign is a choice rather than the product of ignorance.

Awareness alone is not enough. Even a person who knows the law may avoid planning because of fear, procrastination, family difficulty, or a sense that the subject is too remote. Knowledge and the translation of knowledge into action therefore have to be examined together.

Why Relatively Few People Plan Ahead for the End of Life

Avoidance of end-of-life planning does not necessarily reflect irresponsibility. For many people, talking about death feels like inviting disaster, and signing a complex medical document requires imagining frightening and unfamiliar situations. Family members may also shut the conversation down: 'Why are you talking like this? You're healthy.' An attempt to protect the person can thus remove an opportunity for choice.

Another difficulty is uncertainty. A healthy person does not know how he or she will feel if dependent on assistance in the future. Research on adaptation to disability shows that outsiders may judge other people's quality of life as lower than those people report themselves. An advance instruction based only on imagination may therefore become too rigid. Yet without any instruction, decisions may be made by others with no guidance at all.

The solution is not a choice between a detailed document and no document. The approaches can be combined: record values and preferences, appoint a proxy, and specify a few clear limits. This preserves flexibility for future circumstances.

Technical complexity is also discouraging. Long forms, the need for medical explanation, questions about unfamiliar treatments, and periodic renewal create friction. Each requirement is intended to protect the person, but together they can reduce use. This is a classic tension between protection and accessibility.

Digital and language gaps intensify the problem. Online services help those comfortable with digital systems, but an older person, a new immigrant, or a person with a disability may need assistance. A right that can be exercised only through knowledge and technical skill is not fully equal.

The strongest policy approach creates multiple entry points: family medicine, geriatric clinics, oncology, health plans, online services, and community encounters. Advance planning should be a process that can be revisited, not a one-time frightening event.

Postponing end-of-life planning is understandable human behavior. A healthy person prefers to think about work, children, and vacations rather than the possibility of losing capacity. Even someone with chronic illness may see completion of a form as an admission that treatment has failed. A policy that merely places a form on a website assumes the problem is information, when emotional avoidance is also part of the problem.

The moment at which planning is offered matters. Immediately after a serious diagnosis, a person may be overwhelmed; too late, capacity may already be lost. A better approach treats planning as a process rather than an event. A general conversation can be opened, revisited later, and elaborated when the person is ready. This reduces the sense of an ultimatum.

People have difficulty imagining adaptation to future conditions. A healthy person may think that living with a stoma, wheelchair, or dependence would be intolerable and later adapt. Advance directives written without counseling may therefore reflect fear more than an informed preference. The discussion should present possibilities for rehabilitation and adaptation, not only the negative aspects of a scenario.

Family members may encourage planning or prevent it. Some say, 'Don't talk about that,' because of beliefs that discussing death brings bad luck or despair. Others pressure a person to sign. The team's task is to create space in which the individual can speak at his or her own pace. A separate meeting with the family may sometimes help explain that planning is not surrender.

Bureaucracy is a real barrier. Long forms, signatures, medical information, and periods of validity can be discouraging. Each requirement was designed for protection, but the accumulation of requirements can turn protection into an obstacle. Reform should examine which elements are truly necessary to protect free choice and which remain only because of administrative history.

Fear of changing one's mind can also delay planning. People worry that signing will 'lock them in.' It is therefore important to explain that documents can be changed or revoked according to the law and that, while the person has capacity, current wishes are central. A good document is not a trap; it is a backup for a time when the person may no longer be able to speak.

Physicians themselves sometimes postpone the conversation for fear of damaging hope. Palliative practice shows that future planning can be discussed without destroying hope: hope may shift from cure to time with family, comfort, or a personal goal. Avoiding the conversation altogether leaves the person without the opportunity to prepare.

Payment structures also matter. If there is no protected time for a complex discussion, the physician must fit it between other patients. High-quality planning may require half an hour or more. Such investment can prevent later crises and costly unwanted interventions, but the system must recognize it as medical work rather than as an unreimbursed 'conversation.'

At the social level, normalization can change behavior. Like financial estate planning, medical planning can be framed as part of family responsibility rather than as a sign that death is near. A campaign that asks, 'Who will speak for you if you cannot?' may be more accessible than language centered on dying.

The purpose of planning is not to create more refusals of treatment. A person can use it to request treatment as well. Its value lies in clarifying wishes. When this is done early, decisions during a crisis depend less on guessing. Yet even a good document depends on the setting in which the person is treated, which is why the next chapter examines differences between hospital, community care, hospice, and home.

Chapter 11

Implementing the Law in Practice: Hospitals, Community Care, Hospice, Home Care, and the Family in Real Time

Gaps Between Hospitals, Community Care, Hospice, and Home Care

The end of life does not occur in a single place. A person may begin in an oncology ward, go to the emergency department, be discharged home, be hospitalized again, and eventually enter hospice. With each transition the care team changes and sometimes so does the available information. If the patient's wishes do not travel with the patient, every transition becomes a point of risk.

Hospitals are designed for acute care. Their organizational culture tends toward action: test, procedure, intervention. Community care and hospice are built more around continuity and symptom management. This does not mean hospitals cannot provide palliative care, but their structure may create an inertia toward aggressive treatment.

At home, the family becomes a central part of the care system. A decision to remain at home requires team availability, medications, equipment, and a response plan for crises. Without support, a promise of 'dying at home' can become an impossible burden and end in emergency transfer at a difficult moment.

Another gap concerns access to expertise. Dedicated palliative teams are not equally available everywhere or at every hour. When a specialist is unavailable, general teams still need skills in communication, pain management, and end-of-life decision-making. Basic palliative competence should therefore be a cross-cutting clinical skill rather than the preserve of one specialized unit.

Legally, the registry and relevant documents must be accessible at every relevant point of care. A document that remains at home and does not accompany the patient to the emergency department may have no effect in real time. Information infrastructure is therefore part of implementing autonomy.

The real challenge is continuity. The person does not change because he or she has moved from home to hospital; the person's wishes should remain stable even if the system around the person changes.

Hospitals are built to respond to acute conditions, so intervention is often the default. Community care and hospice are more oriented toward continuity and comfort. The same person can therefore encounter a different culture of care depending on the setting. The legal right is supposed to travel with the patient, but its implementation depends on procedures, staffing, and access to information.

In the emergency department, time pressure creates risk. A team that does not know the patient acts under life-saving protocols until contrary information becomes available. If an advance directive or treatment order is not immediately visible, clinicians may begin an intervention the patient did not want. Integration of information systems and clear alerts is therefore critical.

The community setting has the advantage of familiarity. A family physician may know the patient as a person and remember what was said over many years. The disadvantage is availability at night and on weekends. Without accessible palliative support, a family may call an ambulance during a crisis even when the plan was to remain at home. A preference then becomes a hospitalization because no alternative was available.

Hospice offers expertise and presence, but capacity and access may be limited. Waiting lists, eligibility criteria, or distance can undermine equality. A system that recognizes the right to avoid certain treatments must also ask whether it provides a high-quality alternative in the place where the person wants to receive care.

Home care shifts a large amount of work to family members. Changing diapers, administering medication, sleepless nights, and managing equipment can be demanding. It is important not to present 'death at home' as an ideal without asking whether relatives are able and willing to carry the load. They too have limits, and the patient's preference cannot impose an unlimited duty on a family caregiver.

Transitions between institutions are classic failure points. A discharge summary that omits treatment goals, an ambulance crew that receives no information, or a nursing facility unaware of a power of attorney can alter the course of care. Quality standards should therefore require structured transmission of end-of-life information at every transition.

Different teams may also interpret the same terms differently. 'Supportive care' in a hospital may include certain investigations, while in hospice it may mean something else. The plan should describe actions and goals rather than relying on a label. This is especially important for patients who move between settings.

Geographic disparities can remain hidden in raw data. If rates of end-of-life hospitalization are high in peripheral areas, the cause may not be a cultural preference but a shortage of home services. Policy research should connect observed choices to available services before drawing conclusions about what the public wants.

From a legal-liability perspective, a failed transition is often a systems failure. No single person necessarily made a 'negligent decision'; the information simply did not arrive. Such a case requires mapping the system: who was supposed to transmit the information, by what mechanism, and what could actually be seen at the relevant time.

Achieving continuity of care is a condition for the law to mean the same thing in every setting. Otherwise rights depend on the door through which the person enters. Continuity itself also depends on families, which is why the rest of this chapter examines what happens when relatives must make decisions under pressure, sometimes without advance preparation.

Transitions Between Care Settings as a Test of the System

The end of life often unfolds across several settings: home, clinic, emergency department, medical ward, nursing facility, and hospice. At each transition, decisions already made can be lost. A document held by the health plan may not appear immediately in the hospital; a discharge summary may say 'supportive care' without specifying what was decided; an ambulance crew arrives at night and acts on the information available in that moment.

Continuity is not merely the transfer of a medication list. It is the transfer of goals. If the patient wanted to remain at home and avoid repeated hospitalizations, community services must be able to treat dyspnea, pain, and basic crises there. Otherwise the choice exists on paper but disappears at the first moment when the family cannot obtain help.

Geographic and organizational gaps affect the possibility of dying in the preferred place. Home palliative care requires professional availability, medication, equipment, caregiver training, and a response system outside ordinary hours. When one of these elements is missing, a family may call an ambulance even when this was not the original plan. End-of-life choice therefore depends on infrastructure, not only on legal entitlement.

From a legal perspective, transitions sharpen the question of responsibility. Who was supposed to transmit the information, who was supposed to check it, and what could reasonably have been known at the time? An emergency team cannot be expected to follow a document it cannot access, but a system that fails to build an accessible mechanism can fail at the organizational level. This is where patient rights meet system quality.

Differences between care settings become most visible when a family must make decisions in the midst of a crisis. Continuity of care and support for decision-making are therefore two sides of the same implementation problem.

Receiving Information in a Crisis: Time, Memory, and Cognitive Load

A medical crisis changes how people receive information. A relative entering intensive care after sudden deterioration may hear, within minutes, unfamiliar terms, probabilities, possible scenarios, and sometimes a grave prognosis. It is unrealistic to expect a single conversation to be remembered in full. Some information is lost, some acquires a different meaning after a few hours, and a question that seemed clear at noon may return in a different form at night.

The quality of explanation therefore depends on structure as well as content. It is better to begin with the large picture - what has changed, what can realistically be achieved, and the likelihood of returning to the previous condition - and only then move to specific interventions. A list of procedures without a framework can overload rather than clarify. When the family understands the treatment goal, it becomes easier to understand why a particular test is unnecessary or why a time-limited treatment trial is being proposed.

Repeating information is not evidence that the first conversation failed. In end-of-life care, short repeated discussions, updates after clinical changes, and checking understanding by asking relatives to explain in their own words what they understood can all be appropriate. A brief written summary of treatment goals and decision points can reduce discrepancies among family members who heard different parts of the conversation.

Continuity among the professionals speaking with the family matters just as much as the content. When each physician uses different terms, differences in wording may sound like disagreement even when the recommendation is identical. Naming a central professional contact, together with clear documentation of the message that was given, reduces confusion and prevents relatives from having to assemble multiple versions of the situation on their own.

Time also has an emotional dimension. A family may need hours to move from understanding the medical facts to being able to discuss their meaning. This does not mean every decision can be delayed indefinitely, but when there is no immediate urgency, allowing time for processing is part of professional care. The purpose is not to transfer responsibility for the medical decision to the family, but to enable relatives to understand the situation and remain present with the patient without making the conversation itself another source of trauma.

Chapter 12

Why Physicians Find It Difficult to Talk About Death

Physicians are trained to diagnose and treat, but not all receive sufficient training in conversations about prognosis and death. The desire to preserve hope, fear of an emotional reaction, and professional uncertainty can all lead to postponing the discussion. The result is that the patient may hear the information only after the condition has already deteriorated.

Uncertainty is not a reason to avoid the conversation. A physician can say, 'I cannot tell you exactly how much time there is, but I am concerned that we are talking about months rather than years.' This kind of transparency allows planning without pretending that prognosis is precise.

Hope also does not have to remain tied to cure. When oncologic treatment is no longer working, hope can be redirected toward other goals: time with family, control of pain, reaching an important event, or remaining at home. A physician who says, 'There is nothing more we can do,' closes possibilities; a physician who explains what can still be done changes the conversation.

These conversations require recognition of emotion. An immediate numerical answer to the question, 'How much time do I have left?' may miss what the person is really asking: Will I suffer? Will I become dependent? Will I have time to say goodbye? Communication skill is not a humane ornament; it is a tool that makes informed decision-making possible.

There is also an emotional cost to the clinical team. Repeated care of dying patients, conflict with families, and a sense of helplessness can lead to burnout. A system that expects physicians to conduct difficult conversations without support increases the risk of avoidance or emotionally cold communication.

Direct but sensitive language matters. Phrases such as 'the situation is not good' may leave a family without real understanding. It is better to explain what has changed and what is expected, and then allow silence. Not every moment has to be filled with information. People need time to absorb what they have heard.

The physician should also offer a recommendation. A list of options without a professional view can feel like abandonment of responsibility. A physician can say, 'Given what you have told us matters to him and the low likelihood of recovery, I recommend that we do not attempt resuscitation and that we focus on comfort.' The recommendation is transparent and remains open to discussion.

Differences among specialists can be confusing. An oncologist who has known the patient for years may be more optimistic than an intensive care physician who is seeing multi-organ failure. A team discussion before a family meeting can create a coordinated message without erasing genuine professional disagreement.

Simulation-based training can help. Just as clinicians learn cardiopulmonary resuscitation, they can practice communicating prognosis, responding to anger, and discussing DNR decisions. Communication is not merely a personality trait; it is a professional skill that can be improved.

Time pressure is a barrier. A complex conversation squeezed into the end of ward rounds is likely to suffer. An institution that expects good communication must allocate time and an appropriate place for it. Basic privacy matters when a family is receiving difficult information.

A physician must also know how to say, 'I do not know.' Prognosis is uncertain. Credibility increases when the team distinguishes what is known from what is not known and identifies when the situation will be reassessed. False certainty can damage trust when reality changes.

Documentation of a conversation should be factual rather than judgmental. Instead of writing, 'the family is unrealistic,' it is better to record what was explained and what the family is requesting. Judgmental language travels between teams and can shape how people are treated. Professional documentation allows a conversation to continue rather than locking the parties into positions.

The difficulty of talking about death is also connected to legal anxiety. A physician may fear that any statement about futility will be interpreted as giving up, or that any limitation of treatment will create legal exposure. The next chapter examines how defensive medicine can itself harm the patient and how procedural clarity can reduce risk.

Selected research source: Bernacki RE, Block SD. Communication about serious illness care goals: a review and synthesis of best practices. JAMA Internal Medicine. 2014;174(12):1994-2003.

Chapter 13

Defensive Medicine and the Fear of Legal Liability

When the law is unclear to the treating professional, the choice that feels safest personally may be to 'do more.' Additional treatment is sometimes perceived as carrying less legal risk than withholding treatment, even when it has no meaningful medical benefit. This is how defensive medicine can arise at the end of life.

The problem is that more treatment does not always mean more protection for the patient. Aggressive resuscitation, repeated hospitalization, or an invasive procedure can cause suffering without benefit. If fear of liability pushes care toward an intervention that does not fit the patient's goals, the law produces the opposite of what it is meant to protect.

Good protection for the clinical team does not come only from immunity. It comes from a professional process: a clear diagnosis, assessment of capacity, clarification of wishes, a documented conversation, consultation when uncertainty exists, and correct application of the law. High-quality documentation should not be defensive prose filled with generic phrases; it should show the reasoning behind the decision.

Consent also does not 'cover' negligence. A family may agree to an intervention, but if the team fails to provide relevant information or acts below the professional standard, a signature does not erase responsibility. Conversely, a poor outcome does not prove negligence. End-of-life care inherently includes deterioration and death; the question is whether the care and the decision-making were reasonable and appropriately tailored.

This field is especially relevant to lawyers working in medical negligence because the evidence is not limited to laboratory results. It also includes conversations, documents, goals of care, and compliance with required procedures. The distinction between legitimate treatment and a problematic act may depend on how intent and consent were documented.

Defensive medicine occurs when a decision is chosen primarily to reduce legal risk rather than because it is best for the patient. At the end of life, the common defensive direction is continuation: another test, another day of ventilation, another treatment, because not acting appears more dangerous from the perspective of litigation. For the patient, however, continuation itself imposes burdens.

The fear is understandable. Death is irreversible, and a family may later argue that not enough was done. The answer is not to ignore legal risk, but to build a sound process: explanation, documentation, second opinions when appropriate, clarification of wishes, and compliance with the law. A good process offers better protection than purposeless treatment.

Defensive documentation can itself be problematic. Copying stock phrases such as 'all risks were explained' does not prove that a meaningful discussion occurred. The record should be specific to the degree needed: what was discussed, what alternative existed, and what the person decided. Quality is more important than volume.

Defensive medicine can also operate in the opposite direction if an institution is concerned about cost or complications and moves too quickly toward limiting treatment. Legal safeguards must therefore be neutral: they should ensure that decisions rest on expected benefit and the patient's wishes, not on an external incentive.

The distinction between error and negligence matters. A physician may make a reasonable prognostic assessment that later proves wrong. The law does not require prophecy. Negligence examines the process against the knowledge reasonably available at the time. Understanding this distinction can reduce fear of making professional decisions under uncertainty.

Accessible legal consultation within a hospital can help, but it should not turn every conversation into a legal matter. If clinicians are afraid to act without a lawyer, the law has not been successfully implemented. Clear procedures and training should allow most decisions to be handled routinely, with escalation reserved for genuinely complex cases.

A second opinion can reduce risk, but it can also prolong a process if requested automatically. It should be used when it adds value: a disputed prognosis, an unusual decision, or a significant family conflict. Repeating assessments without a clinical reason is another form of defensive practice.

Professional liability insurance and institutional policies shape culture. If physicians receive the message that every complaint is evidence of failure, they may become excessively cautious. A culture of learning, reporting, and review makes it possible to distinguish unavoidable risk from poor practice.

From the patient's perspective, transparency is protective. When the physician explains why a treatment is not recommended and offers an alternative, the decision is less likely to appear arbitrary. A family can disagree and still understand the reasoning. Poor communication is often a greater source of legal conflict than the decision itself.

Defensive medicine also shows that law operates within culture, and culture differs among groups. Trust, religion, language, and history affect how a recommendation is received. A single formulation cannot implement the law effectively across a diverse population.

Medical Negligence at the End of Life: Asking the Right Questions

A claim concerning end-of-life care should not begin with the mere fact that the patient died. Death may have been expected even under optimal care. Legal analysis should break the event into familiar elements: the duty of care, the reasonable standard at the relevant time, whether there was a departure from that standard, whether compensable harm occurred, and whether causation can be established. In this field, possible harm may include not only a shortened life but also an invasive treatment given without valid consent, preventable pain, or an infringement of autonomy.

One distinctive issue is 'negligence through overtreatment.' Law often focuses on harm caused because a necessary act was omitted, but unnecessary action can also cause injury. Resuscitation performed contrary to a valid directive, ventilation initiated without clarifying wishes when there was time to do so, or painful treatment without benefit can raise questions different from the classic claim of delayed diagnosis.

A claim based on defective informed consent also requires precision. The inquiry should identify what information was material to the choice, whether the patient had capacity, who provided the explanation, and what alternative was available. A signed form is not the end of the inquiry. Conversely, a gap in documentation does not automatically prove that no conversation took place; it weakens the ability to establish that it did and creates an evidentiary difficulty.

A lawyer handling medical negligence should therefore read an end-of-life record with both clinical and legal eyes: understand the disease, the decision points, the importance of timing, and the clinical meaning of each intervention. Only then can one ask whether a decision that looks harsh in hindsight was unreasonable at the time. The law should not demand prophecy from physicians, but it may properly demand a professional process, explanation, and documentation.

Chapter 14

Different Populations in Israel: Religious, Haredi, Muslim, Secular, and Immigrant Communities

A single law meets a society that is not uniform. Israel includes communities with different understandings of medical authority, family, religion, and death. A system that assumes one cultural model may misread behavior. A patient who prefers the family to receive information first is not necessarily lacking autonomy; that may be the form of autonomy the patient has chosen. Group identity is a starting point for a question, not an answer about the wishes of a particular person.

In some religious and Haredi communities, a rabbi or other halakhic authority may be an important partner in decision-making. The clinical team's role is not to argue about faith, but to provide accurate medical information that allows a relevant religious ruling. Such cooperation can reduce conflict when it is undertaken with the patient's consent.

Muslim communities may involve similar considerations of religion and family, but no uniform position should be assumed. There are substantial differences within every religious group. Cultural adaptation is not stereotyping; it is the process of finding out what matters to the individual patient.

Immigrants may face language barriers and may be familiar with health systems very different from the Israeli system. Using a child as an interpreter in an end-of-life discussion can be problematic both for accuracy and because of the emotional burden placed on the child. Professional interpretation is part of meaningful informed consent.

The law should protect a person's right to choose a family-centered or religious model of decision-making, as long as that choice is itself free. Autonomy does not require absolute individualism; it also includes the right to say, 'I want my family to make decisions with me.'

Israel is a multicultural society, and it is therefore wrong to assume that every patient wants to make decisions in an individualistic way. Some patients want family members to participate, others seek guidance from a religious authority, and some place the highest value on strict privacy. Adaptation begins with the question, 'How would you like decisions to be made and information to be shared?' rather than with the patient's group affiliation.

In religious and Haredi communities, halakhic guidance may be central. A physician who, with the patient's permission, gives accurate information to a rabbi or halakhic adviser can help the process. Clinicians should not assume in advance that a religious patient will oppose every limitation of treatment. Halakhic distinctions are complex, and the individual's decision may vary.

In Muslim society, extended family and religious belief may play important roles, but again there is no single position. Professional Arabic-language communication and access to religious leaders who understand medical realities can improve discussion. Using a child as the interpreter for a conversation about death is inappropriate when professional interpretation can be obtained.

Immigrants may come from systems in which trust in medicine or in the state was very different. A person who experienced an authoritarian system may fear a form that permits withholding treatment. Explaining that the instrument protects the person's own wishes, and can also express a wish to receive treatment, is important to building trust.

Secular identity is not a single position either. One secular patient may place great value on prolonging life while another prefers to avoid burdensome treatment. Different views can exist within the same family. 'Culture' is therefore never a substitute for listening to the individual.

Language is more than literal translation. Terms such as 'medically futile treatment' or 'terminal' can carry different meanings across languages and communities. A professional interpreter should understand the context, and the physician should use short, clear sentences. Translating a form without adapting the explanation is not enough.

Trust is also affected by inequality. A group that has experienced discrimination within the health system may suspect that a recommendation not to continue treatment reflects a lower value placed on its members' lives. The response is transparency, access to additional opinions, and consistency in professional standards. Equality is not only polite treatment; it also means being able to verify that the same criteria are applied in comparable cases.

Clinical teams need training that prevents stereotyping. Lists such as 'this is how Haredi patients think' or 'this is how Arab families decide' can cause harm. Good training teaches clinicians to ask about values, who should participate, what information is wanted, and which customs matter. It provides tools rather than labels.

End-of-life rituals and customs can affect place, presence, the treatment of the body, and timing. Where they do not conflict with safe care or the law, reasonable accommodation is possible. Such flexibility strengthens trust and reduces the feeling that the health system is taking away not only the patient but also the family's way of saying goodbye.

Israel's diversity reinforces the need for accessible information. If the law is presented only in professional language, people will rely on rumors and partial explanations. The next chapter addresses the gap between the wording of the law and the ordinary citizen's ability to understand and use it.

Cultural Adaptation Without Giving Up Individual Rights

A multicultural society presents a double challenge to the clinical team. On the one hand, understandings of medical authority, family, religion, and death vary across communities and among individuals. On the other hand, cultural knowledge must not be turned into a stereotype. The fact that a patient belongs to a religious community does not by itself tell us what the patient wants; a person may interpret tradition differently from family members or from the community's religious authority.

Language is a central element. Interpretation by a family member may save time but can introduce filtering, especially in discussions of prognosis or refusal of treatment. When the decision is significant, a professional interpreter offers the advantage of allowing the team to check what the patient personally understood. Terms such as 'resuscitation,' 'ventilation,' and 'supportive care' also do not always travel well through direct translation; their meaning must be explained, not merely the words.

Some families ask the team not to disclose the full information to the patient so as 'not to take away hope.' The first step should be to clarify the patient's own preference. Some people want information to be directed to a family member, and that is a legitimate choice; others want to know everything themselves. Respect for culture does not justify automatic concealment from the person whose body and treatment are at issue.

Religious consultation can be meaningful when the patient wants it. Its role is to help the person make a decision within the person's own value system, not to replace the medical or legal process. Appropriate cooperation between religious advisers and the clinical team can reduce conflict, particularly when professional language and halakhic or religious concepts are actually pointing toward the same goal in different words.

Selected research sources: Grove G, Lovell M, Best M. Perspectives of Major World Religions regarding Euthanasia and Assisted Suicide. Journal of Religion and Health. 2022;61:4758-4782; Yang Y et al. Confucian Familism and Shared Decision Making in End-of-Life Care. International Journal of Environmental Research and Public Health. 2022;19.

Chapter 15

Access to Information and the Gap Between the Law and the Ordinary Person

The Dying Patient Law is an area in which legal precision is necessary, but excessive complexity can distance the public. A person should not need a law degree to know how to appoint a health-care proxy. If the official explanation cannot be understood, the right remains most useful to those who are able to navigate or interpret the system for themselves.

Accessibility begins with language: a plain explanation of who qualifies as a dying patient, when a document takes effect, and what it does not authorize. It is especially important to clarify that an advance directive is not 'consent to euthanasia' and that completing one does not prevent ordinary treatment when the person is not in the situation defined by the law.

Accessibility is physical and digital as well. People with visual, hearing, or motor impairments must be able to use the service. An online form that is not accessible, or a process that requires an impossible physical appearance, may disadvantage precisely those for whom advance planning can be especially relevant.

Accessibility must include professionals too. A family physician who is uncertain about the procedure is unlikely to offer it. Short practical training, reminder systems, and clear referral pathways can turn the law from legal material into a clinical tool.

The gap between law and reality is also a measure of regulatory quality. Success is not measured only by the existence of the statute or the absence of violations. It is measured by whether people understand their options, can use them, and whether the health system can actually find and apply their wishes when they are needed.

Access to information begins with language. A legal document can be precise and still be unusable. Citizens need to understand what the law is, what it permits, when it applies, and how to complete the relevant document. One layer of information can present the full legal detail while another provides a plain-language explanation. Simplification is not distortion if it remains faithful to the substance.

A website is important but not sufficient. Older adults, people with limited digital literacy, or those without reliable internet access may remain excluded.

Information should also be available through health plans, hospitals, and community services, as well as through a human help line or service point.

Accessibility for persons with disabilities requires accommodations: screen-reader-compatible documents, large print, sign language, and alternative communication methods. The right to plan ahead cannot depend on the ability to hold a pen or read a conventional form.

Expiration and renewal dates should be accompanied by reminders. Otherwise a registry may contain documents that have expired without the person realizing it. A system that requires citizens to take periodic action should help them remember, especially when the consequence concerns their future wishes.

Information should include clinical examples. Concepts such as mechanical ventilation, DNR, and artificial nutrition are easier to understand through scenarios. At the same time, examples must be presented as illustrations rather than promises; actual decisions depend on the real clinical situation. Videos and physician explanations can supplement written material.

Professional access is part of accessibility too. If a physician cannot find a document in the system during an emergency, the information is functionally inaccessible. Computer interfaces should highlight critical decisions without overwhelming clinicians with alerts.

Information security and privacy matter because these records contain highly sensitive preferences. Broader clinical access must be balanced against protection from unauthorized use. Trust in the registry depends on people knowing who can see the information and what is recorded.

From a policy perspective, the 'user journey' should be measured: how many steps are required from deciding to complete a document through completion, deposit, confirmation, and renewal. Every point at which users drop out reveals a barrier. Usage data can support improvement without changing the underlying legal principles.

The knowledge gap is not only a public problem. A lawyer who does not understand medicine may draft an instruction that cannot be implemented; a physician who does not understand the law may interpret a document incorrectly. Connecting the disciplines is part of professional accessibility.

After examining implementation in Israel, the discussion can move outward to international comparison. The purpose is not to identify an 'advanced country' to copy, but to examine how different systems solve problems of access, eligibility, oversight, and patient choice. Each model will be analyzed according to its structure, not merely by asking whether it permits assisted death.

Accessibility Is Part of Legal Design

A law can be carefully drafted and still remain almost invisible to the citizen. If forms are long, explanations are scattered across websites, and depositing a document requires technical knowledge, the right is used mainly by those who can navigate the system. Accessibility is therefore not merely a matter of customer service. It determines who can turn an abstract right into a practical decision.

Good design begins with language. Alongside the complete legal form, there should be a short explanation that distinguishes advance medical directives, a power of attorney under the Dying Patient Law, and a general enduring power of attorney, and that makes clear when each document comes into effect. Confusion among these mechanisms can lead a person to believe that one instrument was created when legally another was signed.

Digital accessibility alone is not enough. Older populations, persons with disabilities, people who do not speak Hebrew proficiently, and those without convenient computer access need alternative pathways. Telephone support, community assistance, and forms in multiple languages may be more useful than another web page.

The clinical team also needs access. A system that lets a citizen deposit a document but does not display it to the physician in real time creates an illusion of implementation. The service must work as a complete chain: explanation, signature, deposit, retrieval, interpretation, and application. A break in any link can empty the right of meaning at the very moment it is needed.

Chapter 16

Persons with Disabilities and the Fear of Devaluing Life

Few areas of the debate over assisted dying are more charged than its implications for persons with disabilities. The central concern is that society may confuse suffering caused by disease itself with suffering caused by social conditions that can be changed: inaccessibility, loneliness, poverty, lack of personal assistance, untreated pain, unsuitable housing, or absence of family support.

If a person asks to die because home care that would make dignified living possible is unavailable, can the choice truly be described as free? If assisted death is the cheaper and more readily available option for the system, while independent living requires public investment, a serious conflict of interest arises.

At the same time, persons with disabilities should not be treated as incapable of making complex decisions. A paternalistic approach can deny them the very autonomy society grants to others. The challenge is therefore twofold: not to devalue life with disability, while also not presuming that a person lacks decision-making capacity simply because the disability is severe.

A proper assessment should ask not only whether the person understands the decision, but also whether genuine alternatives have been offered. Assisted dying thereby becomes a question of social justice as well as autonomy. Freedom unsupported by realistic opportunities to live with dignity may become an illusory freedom.

Disability advocates sometimes criticize the language of 'death with dignity' when dignity is equated with bodily independence. A person who uses a wheelchair, personal assistance, or mechanical ventilation may live a meaningful life. If the law or a physician assumes that dependence is inherently unbearable, bias may enter the process. Quality of life should therefore be assessed from the person's own perspective, not from the imagination of a healthy observer.

The literature describes a 'disability paradox': people without disabilities sometimes rate life with disability as having a lower quality than do people who actually live with those disabilities. This matters for advance directives and for assisted dying. A decision made in advance may rest on fear that does not match later lived experience. That does not mean advance instructions should be ignored; it means the information offered should not be stereotyped.

Rights organizations also worry about economic incentives. Long-term support is costly; assisted death is comparatively inexpensive. Even if nobody states this openly, the structure of funding can create suspicion. To protect trust, the state should be able to show that the person had genuine access to assistance, housing, equipment, and treatment before death is presented as an option.

Supporters of eligibility respond that denying assisted dying solely because of disability is itself discriminatory. If a person has capacity and meets the relevant legal criteria, why deny a choice available to a person with cancer? Equality may require inclusion as well as protection. The dispute concerns how to identify a wish that is not the product of social failure.

Physicians should also be careful with language. Expressions such as 'confined to a wheelchair' or 'suffers from a wheelchair' can reflect a negative assumption. The wheelchair may be a tool of freedom. Neutral documentation improves decision-making as well: describe what the person can do and what matters to the person, not only deficits.

The distinction between disability and terminal illness must be maintained. A person with a stable disability is not a 'dying patient.' Where disability results from an advancing disease, both dimensions may exist together, but decisions should be based on the disease and the person's wishes, not on a judgment about the value of life with disability.

Accessible communication is itself a safeguard. A person who cannot speak may still have full decision-making capacity. If there is no communication board, assistive technology, or sufficient time, the system may wrongly attribute incapacity and transfer decision-making to others. Technical inaccessibility can thus become a denial of autonomy. Appropriate accommodations should be a condition of any meaningful capacity assessment.

Research on assisted dying should examine who makes requests and why. If patterns of inadequate support emerge, that is a reason to improve services. But it would also be wrong to assume that every request made by a person with a disability is coerced. Paternalism can cause harm just as neglect can.

In Israel, the concern is relevant even without legalized euthanasia. Decisions about ventilation, artificial nutrition, and DNR orders can be influenced by bias about disability. Safeguards should therefore operate within the existing law as well. The question of whose life is considered worth living is not only a future debate.

Concern about social coercion also connects to mental state. Depression and loneliness can change how a person evaluates the future, but they too do not justify automatically removing autonomy. The next chapter separates distress, psychiatric illness, and decision-making capacity.

Selected research sources: Battin MP et al. Journal of Medical Ethics. 2007;33:591-597; Finlay IG, George R. Journal of Medical Ethics. 2011;37:171-174.

Chapter 17

Capacity Under Distress: Depression, Loneliness, Old Age, Poverty, and Family Pressure

Depression, Loneliness, and Whether the Wish to Die Is Always Autonomous

A request to die may express a stable value-based position, but it may also be a symptom. This is one reason why the relationship between end-of-life care and mental health requires particular caution.

Depression can affect hope, appraisal of the future, self-worth, and a person's ability to imagine that circumstances may change. Loneliness can cause a person to see himself or herself as a burden. Anxiety can make the anticipated future appear more threatening than it is. These conditions do not prove that every request to die is pathological, but they do require clinicians to investigate the source of the request rather than merely record it.

The difficulty increases when mental illness itself is the primary source of suffering. Some countries permit assisted dying in certain psychiatric contexts, while others expressly exclude it. The dispute concerns not only the severity of suffering but also prognosis: in a malignant disease, it may sometimes be possible to determine with greater confidence that the medical condition is irreversible. In psychiatry, judging a condition to be "incurable" is more complex, and improvement may remain possible even after years of illness.

Two questions must therefore be separated. Can psychological suffering be as profound and severe as physical suffering? Certainly. But can a system identify with confidence when that psychological suffering can no longer improve? That is a different and much more difficult question.

A wish to die can be a symptom of depression, but not every person who refuses further treatment is depressed. This distinction is fundamental. Automatically pathologizing refusal returns medicine to paternalism. On the other hand, ignoring signs of depression in a terminally ill patient may miss a treatable condition that is affecting the person's wishes.

Mental-state assessment should be focused. Mood, hopelessness, anhedonia, suicidal thinking, cognition, and the ability to understand the decision should be examined. A diagnosis of depression does not necessarily eliminate decision-making capacity; the question is how it affects the particular decision-making process.

Loneliness can itself be profound suffering without constituting a psychiatric diagnosis. A person who has lost social ties and feels burdensome may ask to die because his or her social world has contracted. Social intervention, community support, and volunteers can change that situation. The search for alternatives therefore has to extend beyond medication.

In jurisdictions that permit assisted dying on psychiatric grounds, irreversibility is especially difficult to establish. Mental illnesses can be chronic and treatment-resistant, but uncertainty remains about future treatment and recovery. Canada has repeatedly postponed the application of MAID where mental illness is the sole underlying medical condition, and as of August 2026 the exclusion continues until March 2027. The postponement reflects professional difficulty, not merely political controversy.

Ordinary suicide and medically assisted dying are not classified in the same way in jurisdictions that permit the latter, yet there remains a public question: how can the state invest in suicide prevention in one setting while authorizing an assisted-dying pathway in another? The legal answer rests on eligibility criteria, medical condition, capacity, and voluntariness. Mental-health professionals must nevertheless confront the tension.

Hopelessness is particularly concerning because it can appear rational. A patient may say, "There is nothing in the future," while the medical facts are indeed difficult. Yet treating depression can change the person's appraisal of the future without changing the underlying disease. Recognition is therefore important, especially when the request is new or uncharacteristic.

At the same time, psychiatric assessment can become a barrier if required automatically. Waiting for a specialist may take time, and a terminally ill patient may lose capacity before an assessment occurs. Policy should define when a genuine indication exists. Not every sadness is depression, and not every fear amounts to incapacity.

Loneliness also exposes the public dimension of responsibility. If a person asks to die because there is no caregiver or suitable housing, a fair response first asks whether support can be provided. Choice is not fully free in any meaningful sense when basic alternatives do not exist.

For the clinical team, it is important to ask what a statement means. "I wish I would not wake up" may express pain, a request to talk, or a consistent decision. Immediate psychiatric hospitalization and complete dismissal of the statement can both be wrong. Listening and clarification come first.

The discussion of psychological distress also extends to economics and family life: can old age, poverty, and the cost of care transform an apparently free choice into a decision shaped by a sense of obligation toward others?

Between Depression, Delirium, and Existential Despair

A wish to die in a seriously ill patient requires differential diagnosis. Delirium can arise rapidly because of infection, medication, electrolyte disturbance, or organ failure and can alter decision-making ability from hour to hour. Depression may remain treatable even in advanced disease. Alongside both is despair that is not necessarily a psychiatric disorder. Confusing these states can lead to wrong decisions.

The nurse is often the first person to notice fluctuation: someone who spoke coherently in the morning becomes restless at night, or a wish to die appears mainly during periods of uncontrolled pain. Observation across the day can add information that a single assessment misses. Capacity at the end of life is therefore sometimes a process rather than a stamp.

Legally, the presence of a psychiatric diagnosis does not automatically negate capacity, and its absence does not guarantee it. The question is how the condition affects understanding of information, weighing of that information, and expression of a choice. Where a country's law permits assisted dying in complex situations, the need for consistent professional assessment becomes especially important.

Psychological distress does not arise outside its social context. Loneliness, dependence, old age, poverty, and feeling like a burden on one's family can combine with depression or despair and influence freedom of choice in ways that are difficult to capture in a single decision.

Old Age, Poverty, and the Risk of Financial or Family Pressure

Freedom of choice requires an environment in which a person is allowed to choose life without feeling that doing so harms others. For older people and patients who depend on assistance, that condition is not always present.

A person may say, "I do not want to be a burden," out of love for family. The sentence sounds autonomous, yet it may reflect profound social pressure. If care is expensive, a spouse is exhausted, children are losing workdays, and the state does not provide support services, the decision is being formed within a system of constraints.

Poverty creates a similar problem. A person with resources can purchase private care, adapt a home, obtain additional opinions, and choose a high-quality hospice. A person without those resources may face an institution or isolation. A system that permits assisted dying without ensuring palliative care and basic accessibility risks making social inequality a factor in an irreversible decision.

Protecting autonomy at the end of life therefore does not begin with a request form. It begins with health and welfare policy that reduces external pressure. Only when a person has a reasonable opportunity to live with dignity can a wish not to continue living be examined more fairly.

Old age is not an illness, although it is often accompanied by multiple conditions, dependence, and social loss. Public language that depicts older people as a "burden" is especially dangerous in end-of-life debates. A person may internalize a message that he or she has a duty to die rather than impose on others. Free choice therefore requires a culture in which a person can receive care and support without apologizing for existing.

Poverty changes the range of options. A wealthy person may pay for a home caregiver, adapt housing, and obtain private treatment; a poor person may face institutionalization or loneliness. If both are offered the same legal "choice," their starting positions are not equal. Equality requires examining practical alternatives, not merely the wording of the law.

Family pressure can be explicit or subtle. No threat is required. A person may hear that the children are exhausted and decide that there is no right to continue. It remains that person's decision in one sense, but whether it is truly free is more complicated. An assessment can include a private conversation and the question whether the person would choose differently if adequate support were available.

The cost of care is a public reality and should not be denied. Health systems make decisions about benefit packages and priorities. Yet an individual decision about death should be separated as far as possible from cost-saving considerations. If treatment is not recommended because it offers no meaningful benefit, that should be said. If treatment is not funded, that is an allocation decision and should be transparent.

Inheritance and financial interests raise a classic concern, but most families are not motivated by such interests. Aggressive suspicion can damage trust. A protective mechanism should respond to signs rather than to general suspicion: unusual pressure, inconsistency with the person's known wishes, control over information, or a request that clearly benefits the representative.

Age as an eligibility criterion can itself be discriminatory. Many pathways set a minimum age but no maximum. There is no reason to assume that a request by a ninety-year-old is more or less genuine than a request by a sixty-year-old. Medical condition and decision-making capacity should remain central.

Population aging turns the issue into broad public policy. More people will live with dementia, frailty, and chronic illness. Investment in home care and geriatrics is part of society's answer to end-of-life questions. Law alone is not infrastructure.

Family caregivers also need protection. If they are expected to carry an impossible burden, pressure on the patient may follow. Respite services, financial support, and training protect both sides. A patient's right to live and a caregiver's right not to collapse need not conflict if the state supplies adequate resources.

In jurisdictions that permit assisted dying, data on reasons for requests should be examined in social context. If "being a burden" appears frequently, it is not necessarily proof of coercion, but it is a policy signal. A questionnaire is not enough; qualitative research is needed to understand what the reason means.

Questions of vulnerability become even more difficult when a person is not terminally ill. If natural death is not close, the meaning of assistance is different. The next chapter examines the boundary between severe suffering and a requirement of terminal illness.

Legal safeguards should include review for undue influence while also guarding against paternalism. The fact that a person is poor or old does not eliminate the ability to decide. Good protection does not say, "We will not believe your choice." It says, "We will make sure your options have not been narrowed by a remediable failure."

Selected research sources: Block SD, Billings JA. Patient requests to hasten death: evaluation and management in terminal care. Archives of Internal Medicine. 1994;154(18):2039-2047; Balaguer A et al. An international consensus definition of the wish to hasten death and its related factors. PLoS ONE. 2016; Breitbart W et al. Depression, hopelessness, and desire for hastened death in terminally ill patients with cancer. JAMA. 2000;284:2907-2911; Emanuel EJ et al. Attitudes and desires related to euthanasia and physician-assisted suicide among terminally ill patients. JAMA. 2000;284:2460-2468.

Chapter 18

What Happens When a Person Is Not Terminally Ill but Suffers Severely?

The distinction reflects two different conceptions. Under the first, assisted dying is an exception intended for situations in which death is already near and medicine cannot alter the outcome. Under the second, the central concern is not the amount of life remaining but its quality from the person's own perspective.

Extending eligibility beyond terminal illness creates distinct difficulties. The longer a person's expected lifespan, the more important the possibility of change becomes: a new treatment, adaptation, rehabilitation, support, or a change in living circumstances. A decision that appears reasonable in a moment of crisis may look very different a year later.

On the other hand, a rigid requirement that death be imminent can exclude people who endure very severe conditions for years. This is one of the deepest points of disagreement among models worldwide, and it demonstrates that there is no simple medical line separating "sick enough" from "not sick enough." Ultimately, the boundary is also a value judgment made by society.

Limiting assisted dying to terminal illness rests on an intuition that death is already approaching, so assistance primarily changes its timing and the manner of dying. When a person is not terminally ill, the intervention can shorten life by many years. Some countries therefore use terminal illness as a central moral and legal boundary.

Supporters of broader eligibility argue that suffering is not measured by a clock. A person with a neurological disease or irreversible chronic pain may suffer for years, and sometimes the very duration makes the situation harder. If autonomy and suffering are the justification, proximity to death is not necessarily relevant.

Opponents respond that the longer the horizon, the greater the possibility that treatment, technology, rehabilitation, or adaptation will change the situation. A prognosis of "no improvement" over many years is more difficult than a determination of terminal illness. A higher threshold may therefore be justified.

Canada and Belgium offer comparative material because their systems are not in all cases limited to imminent natural death. Debate around them shows that broader eligibility also changes the professionals whose expertise is needed: more involvement from specialists in chronic disease, psychiatry, and rehabilitation, and less reliance on oncology and hospice alone.

Stable disability is a particularly sensitive case. The fact that there is no cure does not mean that life itself consists of suffering. Physical condition must be separated from the suffering reported by the person. Even then, clinicians must ask whether social support could change the request.

Chronic pain raises a similar difficulty. It can be extremely severe yet fluctuate, and new treatments may emerge. When can it be said that reasonable alternatives have been exhausted? A demand to try "everything" may be unreasonable, but declaring alternatives exhausted too early is also dangerous. There is no simple answer.

Legally, moving from terminal illness to a "serious and irreversible medical condition" greatly broadens discretion. The broader the term, the more protocols, oversight, and case law are needed to reduce inconsistency. Otherwise, two physicians may reach different results in the same circumstances.

Broader eligibility also changes the relationship to suicide. When a person is expected to live for years, the public may find it more difficult to distinguish medically assisted dying from suicide prevention. The legal distinction may rest on illness, capacity, voluntariness, and a regulated process, but it still requires explanation.

Israel chose a framework centered on the dying patient and on withholding or limiting treatment, and it therefore does not currently face a legal pathway for non-terminal suffering. If future reform were opened, one of the first questions would be whether the boundary is proximity to death or the nature of suffering.

The next chapter turns to a situation in which the future may be long but the ability to decide progressively erodes: dementia. There, past wishes, present welfare, and personal identity collide in a way that has no simple solution.

Chapter 19

Hard Cases of Capacity and Protection: Dementia and Minors

Dementia: The Person Who Asked in the Past and the Person Living Now

Dementia creates one of the most difficult dilemmas in the law of advance directives. While still competent, a person may write that if he or she later loses the ability to recognize family members, life-prolonging treatment should not be given. Years later, the person may lack legal capacity yet appear calm, enjoy music, or take pleasure in contact with someone close.

Who is the "real person" for purposes of the decision: the earlier person who planned for the future and expressed a clear wish, or the present person who may no longer understand the condition but still shows preferences and enjoyment?

The problem is less acute when the directive concerns refusal of a particular medical treatment. It becomes especially difficult when a prior document is invoked to justify an active intervention to end life. In that setting, prior autonomy may conflict with present welfare.

Dementia shows that advance directives are not merely a legal technique. They are an attempt to bridge the same person across different points in time. The more irreversible the decision, the greater the need for the document to be clear, current, and based on a genuine understanding of the possible future states.

Dementia also challenges the idea of a one-time decision. A person may write while competent that life in an advanced state would be unacceptable, and later reach that state without remembering the document while appearing content in everyday life. Which self has moral authority - the person who planned the future or the person experiencing the present? There is no agreed answer.

With respect to treatment, an advance directive can guide care even if the person no longer remembers it, but it must be interpreted in context. A request to avoid prolonged ventilation is not necessarily a request to withhold a simple antibiotic that relieves discomfort. The directive must be relevant to the actual decision.

In countries where euthanasia can in some circumstances rest on an advance directive, the difficulty becomes more acute. The intervention is irreversible and the person cannot confirm the wish at the moment it is carried out. Dutch cases have generated debate for precisely this reason. They show that a directive does not solve the problem of identity; it transfers that problem to the physician and the law.

Dementia is not a single uniform pathway. In early stages a person may retain capacity for many decisions; in middle stages capacity may depend on complexity; in advanced stages it may be lost. Diagnosis alone therefore does not eliminate the person's voice. Functional assessment is required.

The current behavior of a person who lacks capacity also matters. The person may physically resist an intervention or show enjoyment. An ethic of dignity requires attention to these responses even when the advance directive provides direction. It is not acceptable to say that the person is "no longer the same person" and may therefore be ignored.

Families carry a heavy burden during prolonged dementia. Exhaustion can influence requests. Support services are therefore a safeguard for the person's wishes, not merely a welfare benefit. When a relative asks to avoid hospitalization, clinicians should understand whether that reflects the person's preference or the collapse of home care.

Artificial nutrition in advanced dementia is a common clinical issue. A feeding tube does not necessarily improve outcomes in every situation, and careful hand feeding may sometimes better serve comfort. Yet food has powerful symbolic meaning. The discussion should present evidence and goals without judging the family.

Dementia sharpens the value of planning ahead, but also its limits. It is useful to record not only interventions but values, and to appoint a proxy who knows the person. Together, these tools allow flexibility when reality differs from the anticipated scenario.

In legal scholarship, dementia is a test of the principle of precedent autonomy: can an earlier wish govern a later self who lacks capacity? The arguments concern identity, interests, and lived experience. Israeli law gives the principle expression mainly in relation to treatment decisions, not euthanasia.

From the person who has lost capacity we move to the person whose capacity is still developing: the minor. Here autonomy is not fully recognized from the outset, yet understanding may be substantial, and parents carry both authority and responsibility. This may be the most sensitive boundary of any end-of-life regime.

Dementia and minority differ medically and legally, but both bring the same underlying question to the center: how should a person's wishes be weighted when capacity is neither simple, stable, nor complete? In dementia, both prior wishes and the interests, behavior, and experience of the person living in the present deserve attention. In minors, developing ability must be combined with protection and parental authority. In both settings, the goal is protection without erasing the person's voice.

Minors and Euthanasia - The Most Difficult Boundary

Minors present a special difficulty because the law recognizes that decision-making ability develops gradually. A young child, a fifteen-year-old adolescent, and a seventeen-year-old are not equivalent in understanding, yet legal systems often need a clear age boundary for irreversible decisions.

In countries that permit some form of assisted dying for minors, the rules are especially stringent and remain highly controversial. The question is not only whether the young person understands that death will occur, but whether he or she can comprehend finality, evaluate alternatives, separate personal wishes from parental influence, and maintain a stable choice under pain and fear.

The role of parents is also complex. They know the child and have a duty of protection. At the same time, they themselves may be grieving, exhausted, and frightened, and are therefore not neutral observers. A legal system must protect both the family and the minor from a decision that arises more from the despair of those around the patient than from the patient's own wishes.

The debate over minors illustrates how difficult it is to convert general values into rules. Autonomy, compassion, and protection of life appear clear in the abstract. In the case of a sick child, they collide with unusual force and without a simple solution.

A minor's understanding of death, illness, and suffering varies by age, development, and experience. An adolescent who has lived with illness for years may understand treatment better than a healthy adult. Chronological age alone is therefore an imperfect measure. Nevertheless, the law uses age because it creates clarity and protects against irreversible decisions during a period of development.

Parents generally make decisions for a child, but their authority is not absolute. They must act in the child's interests, and the state may intervene when refusal of treatment unjustifiably endangers a child. At the end of life, when treatment is no longer curative, the tension is different: how much burden is appropriate, and what weight should be given to the child's wishes?

Belgium and the Netherlands illustrate exceptional models in which some pathways exist for minors under strict conditions. The criteria are demanding and the number of cases small. The very existence of such pathways generates strong opposition because of the difficulty of separating the child's own wish from the influence of parents and clinicians.

Discernment in a minor is not identical to adult capacity. A child may understand pain and death but remain emotionally dependent on parents. Yet dependence does not prove the absence of a personal wish. Assessment requires pediatric expertise rather than simply importing an adult test.

Pediatric palliative care emphasizes family, play, school, and siblings. Goals can differ from those of adults: a day at home or participation in an event may be deeply meaningful. End-of-life conversations should be developmentally appropriate rather than automatically withholding information.

Parents may demand that "everything" be done out of a protective instinct. A team that recommends limiting treatment may be perceived as giving up on a child. Trust is built over time and through continuity of specialists. A decision made in crisis without an established relationship is particularly difficult.

Siblings are often the forgotten group. They experience fear and disruption to family life and may carry guilt. Family-centered care includes them in a developmentally appropriate way. This is not directly a legal issue, but it affects the quality of support surrounding the child.

Constitutionally, children's rights also include a voice appropriate to their development. The issue is not only who signs a form but whether the child is heard. Even when a parent holds formal authority, completely ignoring the child's preferences can violate dignity.

Israel does not permit euthanasia for minors, and the Dying Patient Law contains its own framework of age and authority. Comparison with Belgium is not a proposal for adoption; it is a tool for understanding what conceptual shift would be required to move from a model of limiting treatment to an active model.

Minors expose the boundary of autonomy, but adults also encounter a professional boundary. The next question returns to the physician: is the duty to save life always the supreme purpose of medicine, or does the profession also include acceptance of death?

Selected research sources: Mangino DR et al. Euthanasia and Assisted Suicide of Persons With Dementia in the Netherlands. American Journal of Geriatric Psychiatry. 2020;28:466-477; Groenewoud AS et al. The ethics of euthanasia in dementia. Journal of the American Geriatrics Society. 2022; systematic review on euthanasia in minors, PMID 28573404.

Chapter 20

Reforming Advance Directives and Making the Law Accessible Through Primary Care

After the previous chapters described the law, awareness gaps, and problems of accessibility, the question here is one of design: what should a system look like if it is to translate prior wishes into a reliable clinical tool? The proposed model does not change the boundaries of the Dying Patient Law and does not expand the legal permission to withhold treatment. It concerns the architecture of implementation.

Stage One: Clinical Triggers for Conversation, Not a One-Time Campaign

Instead of relying on a person to initiate completion of a form, the system can identify points at which planning should be offered: diagnosis of an advanced incurable disease, repeated admissions for the same disease, substantial functional decline, initiation of home palliative care, or a transition in which loss of capacity becomes reasonably foreseeable. A trigger does not require a signature. It requires an offer of conversation and an explanation that the decision remains the person's own.

The offer must be separated from the decision itself. An automated system may remind the physician that the topic is relevant, but it should not turn the conversation into a mandatory checkbox. A person may decide not to discuss it at that moment, ask to include a family member, or return to it after consultation. The ability to decline the conversation itself preserves the autonomy of the process.

Stage Two: A Two-Layer Digital Document

The document should contain both a legally precise layer and a clinically readable layer. The legal layer would preserve instructions, signatures, the identity of the proxy, validity dates, and version information. The clinical layer would present in concise form the person's values and goals that can help interpret an unforeseen scenario: what matters most, what degree of dependence the person is willing to accept, what information the person wishes to receive, and who should participate in discussion.

Every change should create a new version rather than erase history. On admission, the team must be able to see clearly which version is valid, when it was prepared, and whether a later version exists. A system that displays several documents without hierarchy increases uncertainty rather than reducing it. Cancellation should also be simple so that a person can change his or her mind without an obsolete instruction remaining active in the system.

Stage Three: Controlled Clinical Activation

Finding a document is not the end of the process. Before implementing it, clinicians must verify that the current clinical situation is one in which the document was intended to operate, that the person cannot currently express an updated wish, and that the instruction is relevant to the scenario. If the patient has capacity, the present conversation takes precedence over interpretation of an older document. If the patient lacks capacity, the document is central evidence but still has to be connected to the medical facts.

If documents conflict with one another, with the proxy, or with the team's interpretation, the system should provide a known escalation route in advance: responsible physician, appropriate consultation, and, where necessary, the institutional committee. The aim is to prevent two opposite failures - ignoring a document because it is complex, and mechanically applying a sentence written years earlier without asking whether it fits the present situation.

Measures of Success: Was the Person's Wish Found in Time, and Did Care Match It?

Reform should be measured by outcomes rather than the number of forms alone. Possible measures include the proportion of people offered a planning conversation at a trigger point; the proportion of documents found during urgent admission; average retrieval time; the proportion of cases involving conflicting versions; the number of committee referrals caused by ambiguity; and whether care matched documented preferences when that could reasonably be determined.

Equity should also be measured. A digital system that works well for Hebrew-speaking users in central Israel may fail an older person, an Arabic- or Russian-speaking patient, a person with visual impairment, or someone who does not use a smartphone. Implementation must therefore include human assistance, accessible documents, translation, and monitoring of differences among regions and population groups.

Finally, change should be introduced in stages. A pilot in several health plans and hospitals can reveal which triggers generate too many alerts, which wording is poorly understood, and what happens during transfers between institutions. Only after measurement and correction should the model be expanded. The advantage of this approach is that it strengthens rights that already exist without turning every operational improvement into a renewed debate over whether euthanasia should be legalized.

Chapter 21

Should Israel Reconsider Medically Assisted Dying?

The question whether Israel should reopen the debate on medically assisted dying does not require a predetermined yes or no. The discussion itself may be legitimate after years of experience with the existing law and in light of changes elsewhere in the world.

The case for reconsideration rests on autonomy, the accumulated experience of countries that have built oversight mechanisms, and cases in which palliative care does not reduce suffering to a level the patient considers acceptable. Supporters of renewed review may argue that Israeli society can examine a very narrow option without necessarily adopting the broadest international models.

The case against rests on the sanctity of life, Israel's religious and social characteristics, concern for harm to vulnerable people, and the possibility that an already strained health system is not the ideal setting in which to add a pathway where death is a planned outcome. Opponents may also argue that Israel's central problem is not lack of an option to die, but unequal and inconsistent access to palliative care and advance planning.

A responsible public debate would need to avoid two extremes: presenting every form of assistance in dying as murder, or portraying every objection as cruelty. A democratic society can disagree profoundly and still examine evidence, models, and consequences without degrading those who hold different positions.

Reconsideration does not mean change. A society can review a law and decide to leave it in place. The discussion itself can be healthy if based on facts rather than fear. Since 2005, more jurisdictions have introduced pathways and more data have accumulated. Israeli society has also changed. It is therefore reasonable to ask whether the balance still reflects the public and the professions.

The first step is to define the question. "Euthanasia" is too broad. Is the proposal physician-assisted self-administration for a competent terminally ill adult only? Administration by a physician? What about residency, psychiatric illness, dementia, and minors? Without definition, opposing camps may be arguing about different things.

A new public committee could include physicians, nurses, lawyers, persons with disabilities, representatives of religious communities, palliative-care clinicians, mental-health professionals, and members of the public. Representation is not decoration; it prevents experts from speaking on behalf of groups they do not know.

Israeli data should be collected on use of advance directives, palliative care, public attitudes, professional attitudes, and cases that reach formal dispute. If the principal problem is failure to implement the existing law, opening a new boundary may not be the answer.

Comparative law can present several models rather than a single template. A narrow American model differs from Canada; the Netherlands differs from Switzerland. Any committee should ask which safeguards fit the Israeli system.

Religion and tradition will form part of the debate, but a democratic state also includes citizens who do not accept religious authority. Any compromise should be expressed in a public language understandable to all, even if its sources are diverse.

Persons with disabilities should be at the center. A right to die cannot be discussed without demonstrating how the state secures a right to live with support. Any proposal should include an impact assessment concerning vulnerable populations.

Professionals must also say whether they are prepared to participate. A law with no one willing or trained to implement it will create a crisis. Conscience, training, oversight, and professional liability all require examination.

The debate should be slow enough to be serious without continuing indefinitely. An options paper could be published, public comments invited, and open hearings held. Transparency improves legitimacy even if the final outcome is retention of the existing prohibition.

For purposes of this book, there is no need to choose an answer. The conclusion is that any future debate must begin from the distinctions already developed. "Compassion" is not a statutory provision, and "sanctity" is not an implementation mechanism. If change is chosen, the details must be designed. But substantial reform is also possible without legalizing euthanasia at all.

Four Threshold Conditions Before Changing the Israeli Boundary

First, the model must be defined precisely. It must be clear whether discussion concerns only terminally ill patients, whether self-administration is required, and how dementia, psychiatric illness, and minors are treated. Each of these choices changes the nature of the regime more than the general label "euthanasia."

Second, genuine and accessible alternatives are required. A safeguard stating that "alternatives are available" is meaningless if palliative care, mental-health treatment, home nursing, or support for a person with disability are not equally accessible. Before creating an irreversible option, the state should be able to show that the choice is not the product of a remediable lack of care.

Third, professional roles and conscience must be defined. The law would need to determine who assesses capacity, who performs or supplies the intervention, what the nurse's role is, how conscientious objection is handled, and what duty the institution bears to ensure continuity. A framework centered only on the requesting patient and ignoring the clinical team will struggle to operate safely and legitimately.

Fourth, oversight and data requirements should be established in advance. If society changes such a fundamental boundary, it should agree before implementation on what must be reported, who reviews cases, which deviations will be investigated, and what data will be published. Future debate about success, equity, or a "slippery slope" will be weak without an evidentiary infrastructure capable of testing those claims.

Chapter 22

An Israeli Model for Reform: Improving End-of-Life Care Without Necessarily Crossing the Boundary Into Euthanasia

From Diagnosis to Architecture

The previous chapters have already identified the difficulties: limited use of advance directives, accessibility gaps, prognostic uncertainty, variation among institutions, the need for available palliative care, and disputes that sometimes reach formal mechanisms too late. The purpose of this chapter is neither to repeat those problems nor to explain the forms again. It proposes a system architecture in which each component addresses a different failure, while preserving the possibility of deep reform even if Israel's prohibition on active euthanasia and assisted suicide remains unchanged.

The starting point is that end-of-life reform is not an amendment to one section of a statute. A good decision depends on a chain: early identification of a person whose illness is advancing; a conversation before crisis; a document that can be found in time; real palliative care; a team that knows the law; a rapid mechanism for disputes; and data that allow the system to learn from implementation. If one link is missing, a written right can remain powerless at the bedside.

Component One - Clear National Governance and a Single Professional Address

The system needs clear institutional ownership of implementation of the Dying Patient Law. It is not enough for forms to sit in a registry and committees to exist in the statute. The Ministry of Health should consider a national unit responsible for implementation indicators, training, publication of updated guidance, analysis of recurring disputes, and coordination among hospitals, health plans, Magen David Adom, hospices, and long-term-care institutions. Its role would not be to decide in place of the responsible physician, but to ensure that the system speaks one language.

The unit could publish a uniform annual report: how many valid advance directives and powers of attorney exist in the registry; how many were actually retrieved during a relevant admission; how many matters reached committees; response times; recurrent categories of dispute; and regional availability of palliative services. Transparency would then become a tool for improvement rather than merely a response to later information requests.

Component Two - Advance Planning as a Clinical Pathway, Not an Occasional Form

The digital model and the connection to primary care proposed in Chapter 20 should be one layer within the broader reform rather than the entire project. The online service and national registry currently operated by the Ministry of Health are important infrastructure, but success should be measured not by the number of files deposited but by whether the person's wishes are found and understood when a clinical decision is required. Advance planning should therefore be linked to clear clinical triggers: diagnosis of advanced disease, recurrent admissions, substantial functional decline, initiation of a treatment with long-term consequences, or transition to a long-term-care setting.

At none of these points must a person be required to sign immediately. The process can begin with a goals-of-care conversation and documentation of values and communication preferences. The legal document may follow. This avoids introducing advance directives for the first time in a crisis while also avoiding forced conversations about death at every routine visit.

Component Three - A Goals-of-Care Document That Travels With the Patient

An advance directive alone does not solve the problem of transitions among community care, ambulance, emergency department, hospital ward, and hospice. Alongside it, there should be a short, current clinical document summarizing present goals of care: the medical condition, who makes decisions, which treatments fit the goals, whether a DNR order exists, and what should occur if the patient's condition deteriorates. This is a working clinical document, not a substitute for the legal directive.

Its advantage is reduced loss of information. When a patient is transferred to hospital at night, a new team should not have to reconstruct within minutes a conversation that took months. The document should be accessible in the electronic record and updated when goals change. It also narrows the gap between a general decision and its execution: the words "supportive care" are not enough if an emergency team does not know whether to give antibiotics, fluids, oxygen, or transfer the patient to intensive care.

Component Four - A Practical Right to Palliative Care in Every Setting

End-of-life law without palliative services creates an illusory choice. A person may formally choose to avoid life-prolonging treatment, but if the alternative is pain, breathlessness, anxiety, or absence of support at home, the person is not choosing between two reasonable options. The Ministry of Health currently notes that palliative care is available in the community and that health plans can provide home hospice. Reform should turn that principle into a standard of availability rather than an option dependent on geography or a family's ability to navigate the system.

The target should include response times, telephone consultation outside regular hours, rapid access to medications for symptom relief, home visits, and orderly transitions between home and inpatient care as needs change. Palliative care is not a "final stage" that starts only after every other treatment stops; it is a layer of care that can begin earlier and grow as disease progresses.

Component Five - Rapid Dispute Resolution Before Conflict Becomes a Crisis

The committees established by law are important, but in a field where decisions are measured in hours and days, operational accessibility is also required. The proposed model is a network of readily available institutional consultation with an expedited route for disputes that cannot wait for a scheduled meeting. Not every question needs a full formal committee hearing; in many cases, consultation with a senior physician, palliative specialist, lawyer, or ethicist can resolve misunderstanding before it hardens into confrontation.

For more complex disputes, multidisciplinary composition and documentation should be preserved. The committee should ask questions in a consistent order: What are the medical facts? What is known about the patient's wishes? What authority does each participant have? What alternatives exist? Which values are genuinely in conflict? A fixed structure reduces the risk that a value dispute will hide behind a medical assertion, or the reverse.

Component Six - Re-examining the Continuous-versus-Cyclical Distinction Without Jumping to Euthanasia

Difficulty with the distinction between continuous and cyclical treatment does not force a binary choice between leaving the law untouched and permitting withdrawal of every treatment. A focused professional review can examine settings in which technology has changed since 2005. One option is wider use of time-limited treatment trials: treatment begins under agreed conditions, goals and a reassessment point are defined in advance, and the fear that agreement to a trial will become an irreversible commitment is reduced.

Another option is to examine technological and procedural solutions that allow planned cessation in accordance with the law, using controlled pilots and evaluation of outcomes. The idea is not to evade the legal boundary, but to ask whether tools created two decades ago still produce the result the legislature intended: respect for wishes without turning clinicians into performers of an act whose purpose is death.

Component Seven - Protection of Vulnerable Patients as a Condition of Autonomy

A reform that strengthens the power of individual choice must invest equally in the conditions that make choice free. Interpreters, communication accommodations for persons with disabilities, assessment of delirium or depression when relevant, identification of family or financial pressure, and social assistance when a request to limit treatment rests on a sense of burden are all required. Protection is not intended to cancel the choice of a vulnerable person; it is intended to ensure that vulnerability is not speaking in the person's place.

Accessibility itself should be measured. An online form that a blind person cannot complete, a conversation without an interpreter, or a system that assumes everyone can type and sign digitally creates discrimination inside a mechanism designed to protect autonomy. Implementation metrics should therefore measure not only how many people use the system but also who remains outside it.

Component Eight - Joint Training for Medicine, Nursing, Law, and Social Work

End-of-life training should be case-based. A lecture on statutory sections does not teach a physician how to tell a family that CPR will not achieve the outcome they imagine; it does not teach a nurse what to do when a patient appears to have changed his or her mind; and it does not teach a lawyer how to read a medical record in which "the patient lacks capacity" was written without supporting assessment. Multidisciplinary simulation can create a common language and expose points of failure before they occur in a real patient.

Training should recur throughout professional careers. Changes in technology, policy, and case law make one-time instruction insufficient. Community, emergency, and intensive-care teams are especially important because they make decisions under pressure and may have only partial information about earlier wishes.

Component Nine - Measuring Concordance With Wishes, Not Only Procedural Compliance

A system may be excellent at completing forms and still miss the law's purpose. The central measure should be whether care, insofar as it can be determined, matched the person's wishes and the goals agreed with that person. Alongside metrics such as committee response times, number of documents, and rates of palliative consultation, the system should examine how often a directive was found in time, how often discovery of a document changed the plan, and how many inter-institutional transfers occurred without goals of care being transmitted.

Data should be anonymized and privacy protected, but public at a level that permits scrutiny. The purpose is not simplistic ranking of hospitals but identification of patterns. A hospital with almost no committee referrals may truly have few disputes, but it may also be a hospital where the mechanism is not understood. Numbers need context.

Component Ten - A Mechanism for Periodic Review of the Law

Technology and society change faster than legislation. It would therefore be appropriate to establish periodic review, for example every five years, examining definitions, use of legal mechanisms, development of palliative care, and international experience. Review does not require amendment; a reasoned decision to retain an existing rule can itself be an outcome. The advantage is that the law does not become immune to updating merely because it once embodied a historic compromise.

Order of Implementation - What Can Be Done Before Legislative Change

A substantial part of this model does not require amendment of the criminal prohibition, or even immediate amendment of the Dying Patient Law. The first stage can improve digital infrastructure, training, metrics, coordination among settings, and palliative availability. The second can strengthen dispute-resolution mechanisms and pilot goals-of-care planning and documents. Only in a third stage, after the system has accumulated data, is there a basis for considering amendments to definitions or classifications of treatment. This sequencing distinguishes failure of the law from failure of implementation.

A staged reform also has a public advantage. Debate over euthanasia tends to dominate every discussion of end-of-life care even though most end-of-life decisions do not concern euthanasia. A stronger system can improve the lives of patients and families now without waiting for national agreement on the most fundamental question. If Israel later decides to reconsider medically assisted dying, the debate would then take place within a system capable of providing palliative care, identifying wishes, detecting vulnerability, and publishing data - rather than against a background of service gaps masquerading as value choices.

An Additional Component - Funding and Incentives Aligned With Reform Goals

Behavior in a health system does not change through a circular or website alone. If a goals-of-care conversation requires an hour but is funded as though it were a brief visit, and if a palliative home visit is harder to organize than hospital admission, the system will continue to favor the operationally easier pathway even when it is less appropriate for the patient. Reform should therefore include incentives: protected time for complex conversations, funding for community services, staffing for palliative consultation, and recognition of coordination work that is not a procedure but can prevent admissions and conflict.

Funding must also avoid dangerous incentives. An institution should not profit directly from reducing treatment for an individual patient, because that can undermine trust and introduce financial considerations into a setting where the patient needs to know that the recommendation was made for his or her benefit. It is preferable to reward process and quality - availability of palliative care, documentation of goals, retrieval of directives, committee response times - rather than outcomes such as fewer hospital days or a higher proportion of DNR orders.

Learning Regulation Rather Than One-Time Reform

End-of-life care is especially suitable for a learning-regulation model. Rather than wait a decade for a major statutory amendment, several hospitals and health plans can pilot a goals-of-care document, rapid consultation service, or advance-planning model, measure outcomes, and correct problems before national expansion. A good pilot should also examine unintended effects: Did the conversation increase anxiety? Did some populations use the service less? Did clinicians understand the difference between a clinical document and a legal directive? Did a new burden simply move elsewhere in the system?

This approach allows reform to be built without assuming that every idea that sounds correct will work identically in every institution. Israel's health system is diverse: a large tertiary hospital in the center, a peripheral clinic, a long-term-care institution, and home hospice operate under different conditions. Learning regulation permits uniform principles while adapting the route to them to local reality.

What About People Who Do Not Meet the Six-Month Definition?

A reform model cannot assume that every end-of-life decision occurs within the Dying Patient Law. People with dementia, neurological disease, heart failure, or other chronic conditions can face profound treatment decisions long before physicians can estimate that life expectancy is no more than six months. They require the general tools of the Patients' Rights Law, informed consent, an appropriate power of attorney, and goals-of-care planning even before the specific mechanisms of the Dying Patient Law are activated.

The proposed reform should therefore build a continuum rather than a gate. Goals-of-care conversations and advance planning can begin because of clinical need without granting a legal status that does not yet exist. When the statutory definition is later met, the documents and discussions can connect to the specialized framework. This prevents postponing an important conversation merely because prognosis is still too long, while preserving the distinction between general patient rights and the special regime for the dying patient.

This continuum is especially important in dementia. If the system waits until the person has already lost capacity before asking what he or she wanted, the opportunity has closed. Advance planning need not decide every future intervention, but it allows a person to describe values, appoint a representative, and explain what matters before disease restricts the ability to do so. Reform can thus strengthen autonomy without changing the six-month definition itself.

Part Four

The World Confronts the End of Life - and What Israel Can Learn From It

Chapter 1

Permissive Europe - The Netherlands and Belgium: Established Models, Autonomy, and Oversight

The Dutch model is important because it did not appear overnight in a statute legalizing euthanasia. Over many years, Dutch practice developed through case law, professional guidance, and prosecutorial policy before receiving statutory form. That history affects how the system operates: the law did not create a medical culture from nothing, but converted gradually developed criteria into a supervised pathway. Copying statutory language without the surrounding professional culture and institutions may therefore miss the substance of the model.

In the Netherlands, euthanasia and assisted suicide remain offenses in principle, but a physician can avoid criminal liability when the statutory due-care criteria are satisfied and the case is reported as required. The structure matters. This is not a general permission for anyone to cause death; it is a conditional professional exception. The physician must be satisfied, among other things, that the request is voluntary and well considered, that suffering is unbearable with no prospect of improvement, that the patient is informed, that there is no reasonable alternative, that an independent consultation has occurred, and that the procedure is performed with due medical care.

The criteria are not mechanical. "Unbearable suffering" contains a personal dimension, yet the physician must be able to ground the assessment in a medical condition. "No prospect of improvement" requires inquiry into alternatives. The model therefore does not rest on autonomy alone; a request does not automatically create a right to euthanasia. The Dutch government emphasizes that patients cannot compel physicians to perform it, and physicians may refuse. The model preserves tension between personal choice and professional responsibility.

Review generally occurs after the act through regional review committees that receive reports and assess compliance with the due-care criteria. Ex post review allows a physician to act at the appropriate clinical time without awaiting a judicial order in every case, but it requires full transparency because the act is irreversible. Where a committee concludes that the criteria were not met, the matter may be referred to the competent authorities. The model thus relies on professional trust backed by oversight rather than on trust without review.

Minors illustrate the boundaries of the model. Dutch law permits requests from certain ages under demanding conditions and with defined parental involvement, making it broader than systems that restrict assisted dying to adults. The existence of the legal route does not mean the practice is routine; it raises difficult questions about developing capacity, parental authority, and assessment of suffering. Comparative analysis must distinguish existence of a legal route from frequency of use.

Advance directives can also play a role in the euthanasia context, a matter of particular sensitivity in dementia. The difficulty is interpretive: a document written while the person had capacity may be invoked when the person can no longer confirm the wish. Such cases have generated legal and professional controversy in the Netherlands. They demonstrate that "future autonomy" is more complicated when the act is euthanasia rather than withholding treatment.

The Dutch model also separates euthanasia from palliative treatment. Palliative sedation is not classified as euthanasia when its purpose is relief and death results from the underlying disease. This distinction is essential for data. Treating every sedation as "assisted death" artificially inflates numbers and conflates different interventions. Reliable reporting requires consistent definitions.

In Israeli debate, the Netherlands is often used as a symbol - positive or negative - rather than studied as a legal system. Supporters cite it as evidence that regulation is possible; opponents cite concern over widening boundaries. Serious research must move from symbol to data: what categories exist, how committees operate, what deviations occur, and what has changed over time. Only then can claims about a slippery slope or regulatory stability be examined.

The lesson for Israel is not necessarily to adopt or reject the Dutch model. It is that a system permitting intentional life-ending action requires mature reporting, consultation, training, and review mechanisms. It also requires clear answers about physician conscience and complex cases such as psychiatry and dementia. If a society is not prepared to answer those questions, a general declaration of autonomy is not enough.

As of August 2026, the Dutch framework remains one of the oldest and best documented in the world. Its longevity makes it an especially valuable laboratory: not only how a law begins, but how it is interpreted, how oversight develops, and how boundaries are tested after years of practice. Belgium adopted a related but non-identical model and has been particularly important in debate over minors.

How to Compare Legal Systems Without Distorting Them

Serious international comparison begins by defining the unit of comparison. "Euthanasia" is not sufficient because one jurisdiction permits administration by a physician, another permits only medication self-administered by the patient, and a third prohibits both while recognizing a broad right to refuse treatment. Each system should therefore be broken down by eligibility, type of act, person who performs it, procedure, oversight, and available alternatives.

Sources must also be distinguished. A statute enacted by parliament, a constitutional judgment, a Ministry of Health procedure, and a professional guideline do not have the same legal status. In federal systems, rules may differ among subnational units. Academic work should identify the date of legal verification because the field changes quickly and a bill can become law - or fail - between manuscript preparation and publication.

Good comparison does not rank countries along a moral scale. It asks what problem each arrangement sought to solve and what safeguards it created. Usage data matter, but they must be interpreted in light of population size, service structure, and reporting definitions. A higher number is not necessarily evidence of regulatory failure, and a lower number is not necessarily evidence of better protection.

The Dutch Lesson: Professionalism Is Tested Even After a Request Is Accepted

The most revealing stage of the Dutch model begins after the patient has expressed a request. The physician must distinguish a stable wish from a statement born of crisis, examine reasonable alternatives for relief, and obtain independent consultation. Clinically, assessment of suffering cannot be reduced to asking how much the patient hurts. Physical, psychological, and social dimensions must be explored, and the patient must understand the situation.

The medical record is crucial. In a system reviewed after the act, the record must allow the committee to reconstruct the decision-making process: when the request emerged, whether and how it was repeated, what alternatives were offered, what the independent consultant concluded, and how the possibility of withdrawal of the request was preserved. Such documentation should not be a ritual of legal self-protection; it is the means by which the quality of an irreversible decision becomes reviewable.

Cases involving dementia or psychiatric illness show that the model is not an "autonomy-only" test. The more difficult it is to assess capacity, stability of wishes, or prospects for improvement, the greater the professional responsibility. This is also where staff members who know the patient over time become especially important: changes in behavior, fluctuations in wishes, or response to treatment may all be relevant.

For Israeli discussion, the main contribution of the Netherlands is methodological. Learning from the model requires more than counting cases. One must examine consultation quality, diagnostic categories, reporting processes, and the reasoning published by review committees. Only then can one ask whether boundaries have expanded, tightened, or whether the system has simply become better at identifying and reporting situations that previously existed.

Belgium - Autonomy, Suffering, and Extension of the Law to Minors

Belgium legalized euthanasia in 2002, around the same period in which the Netherlands formalized its pathway. The similarities often cause the two to be treated as one model, but there are differences in conditions, oversight, and later developments. Belgium is particularly important because the law was extended to minors under stringent conditions, placing it at the center of debate about the limits of autonomy at a young age.

The Belgian framework requires a voluntary, considered, and repeated request, a serious and incurable medical condition, and constant and unbearable suffering resulting from that condition. The procedure differs according to whether death is expected in the near term. Where the patient is not terminal in the sense of imminent death, additional requirements and a waiting period apply. The structure shows that a state can recognize severe suffering outside a short terminal window while adding safeguards as the connection to natural death becomes more remote.

A physician is not obliged to perform euthanasia. Conscientious refusal is preserved, while duties regarding information and continuity apply under the law. This balance recognizes the service as lawful without turning every physician into a performer of the act. In practice, access also depends on availability of professionals willing to participate, so conscience is not merely an individual right but an element of system design.

The extension to minors does not rest on a numerical age threshold alone, but on the minor's capacity for discernment and understanding, a serious medical condition and suffering, parental involvement, and other safeguards. The pathway is very narrow and cases are rare. Its existence nonetheless poses a basic question: if an adolescent understands illness and death, should age alone exclude every option; and conversely, can a system ensure that a minor's decision is not shaped by dependence on parents and clinicians?

Official figures illustrate how exceptional the pathway for minors is. In 2025, Belgium reported one case involving a minor, bringing the cumulative number to seven since the 2014 extension of the law to minors. The figure does not resolve the ethical dispute, but it distinguishes the existence of legal authority from frequency of use.

Belgium also illustrates the difference between euthanasia and withdrawal of treatment. According to official information, discontinuing unwanted or futile treatment is not classified as euthanasia, and palliative sedation is a separate category. The distinction improves data accuracy and prevents every death following a treatment decision from being treated as the same act.

Oversight is conducted by a federal commission that receives reports and reviews compliance with legal conditions. Such a system allows data to accumulate and trends to be monitored. Ex post review, however, depends on the quality and completeness of reporting. A case not reported, or classified under a different category, will not appear in the same dataset. Official data are therefore important but must be read within the method by which they are collected.

The official report for 2025 stated that the commission received and examined 4,486 registration forms, representing approximately four percent of all deaths in Belgium that year. The commission reported that none of the reviewed reports was referred to the public prosecutor. Figures of this kind allow monitoring of scale, but they cannot be interpreted without understanding reporting mechanisms and categories.

Belgian debate also includes psychiatric illness and non-terminal conditions, an area that attracts considerable criticism. Determining that there is "no reasonable prospect of improvement" is particularly difficult in psychiatry, where a long course of illness, the therapeutic relationship, and future innovations may change the picture. Supporters emphasize equality of suffering; opponents emphasize uncertainty of prediction and the effect of illness on wishes. Israel can learn mainly about the difficulty of defining a threshold, not from any ready-made answer.

From a disability-rights perspective, the model raises the question of how to ensure that a request is not the product of absent support. Formal freedom is insufficient if a person asks to die because accessible housing or assistance is unavailable. Evaluation of alternatives must therefore include treatment and social support, not medication alone. This issue will recur in the normative discussion.

For an Israeli physician, Belgium sharpens what is different at home: Israel has no lawful pathway for an intentional act designed to cause death, even when suffering is severe and the request persistent. The difference is not simply a form; it reflects a different conception of the physician's role. Both systems, however, attribute importance to palliative care, patient wishes, and documentation.

Belgium and the Netherlands are therefore similar but not identical. Comparing them shows why the phrase "Europe permits" is inadequate. Europe itself contains diverse approaches. Luxembourg and Spain add models of explicit legislation with their own characteristics, illustrating how newer laws can draw on the experience of earlier jurisdictions.

Chapter 2

Europe Beyond the Netherlands and Belgium - Luxembourg, Spain, Switzerland, Germany, Italy, France, and the United Kingdom

Luxembourg and Spain - Explicit European Legislation and the Challenge After Enactment

Luxembourg is a small country, but it is important in comparative law because it is among the European jurisdictions that established by statute pathways for euthanasia and assisted suicide. The size of its health system may permit forms of coordination and oversight that differ from those available in a larger state, so direct conclusions for Israel require caution. It nevertheless demonstrates how a legal system can distinguish the general criminal prohibition from a conditional medical exception.

The Luxembourg framework, like neighboring systems, is built around a voluntary request, a serious medical condition, and unbearable suffering, together with duties of consultation and documentation. The comparison matters less for the wording of individual provisions than for the structure: the law does not say in general that "a person may die"; it specifies who may act, under what conditions, and through what review procedure. Liberty is translated into a legal pathway with gates.

Spain adopted Organic Law 3/2021 and created a regulated prestación de ayuda para morir within the health system. The choice of an organic law and integration of the service into the public system give the arrangement the character of a regulated health entitlement rather than merely a criminal-law defense for the physician. Institutionally, this differs from a model in which the act remains only an exception to an offense.

The Spanish process includes requests, assessments, and review through designated bodies. Its structure seeks review before performance rather than relying exclusively on after-the-fact reporting. A possible advantage is prevention of error before an irreversible act; a possible disadvantage is delay and bureaucratic burden for a person in distress. Comparison with the Netherlands illustrates two different philosophies of oversight: more prior authorization versus more retrospective review.

Spain also illustrates implementation in a country with autonomous regions and varying health systems. A national right can encounter local differences in availability, training, and conscientious objection. The lesson for Israel is straightforward: national legislation does not guarantee uniformity among hospitals, health plans, and peripheral regions. Implementation must measure the path from legal right to actual service.

Conscientious objection has an institutional place in Spain, requiring a balance between the professional's conscience and patient access. When the state defines a service as part of health care, it must plan how the service will remain available where some staff object. Mechanisms may include registration or referral arrangements, but each raises questions of privacy and possible stigma for professionals.

Luxembourg and Spain also show that the word "Europe" conceals different legal traditions. A historically Catholic country can adopt a model different from a Protestant one, and there is no simple correlation between public religion and legislation. Change can arise from social movements, judicial decisions, political coalitions, and clinical experience.

For newer systems, data require time to stabilize. Early years involve professional learning, development of procedures, and changes in interpretation. Comparing case numbers in Spain after only a few years with the Netherlands after decades would therefore be misleading unless the stage of development is taken into account.

Spain is especially interesting for Israel because it offers an example of a pathway embedded in a public health system, while Israel has kept intentional life-ending action outside permitted medical practice. The issue is not only differing values but also what the state is prepared to require from the health system: committees, response times, training, and workforce planning.

The wider European map shows that change is not uniform. Switzerland has a different tradition of assisted suicide without a classic euthanasia model, while Germany, Italy, France, and the United Kingdom remain on distinct legal and political paths. These "intermediate" jurisdictions often teach more about regulatory diversity than a simple comparison between full permission and full prohibition.

Luxembourg and Spain demonstrate that permission acquires practical meaning only through institutions. Spain created guarantee and evaluation commissions as part of the process, alongside a mechanism for conscientious objection. The design seeks protection in two directions: of the applicant from the personal barrier of a single clinician, and of the clinician from being required to perform an act contrary to conscience.

From a health-system perspective, conscientious objection is not only a private matter. If most professionals in a region object, a legal entitlement can become inaccessible in practice. Conversely, forcing a clinician to perform an irreversible act can harm both the professional and the profession. A workable regime therefore has to address staffing, referral, and continuity, not merely declare the two rights.

Spain also illustrates the role of constitutional review. Enactment by parliament does not end debate about the right to life, autonomy, or the public duty to protect vulnerable people. Constitutional review is not necessarily opposition to the law; it is a means of testing whether the pathway, safeguards, and balances fit the foundational principles of the legal system.

Clinically, legal access to assisted dying does not reduce the need for palliative medicine. If anything, it increases the need to demonstrate that the patient understands available measures for relief and is not choosing death because the system failed to provide basic care. Law, financing, and health services meet at this point: a right on paper depends on the quality of alternatives in reality.

Europe contains no single model. Alongside explicit legislation are frameworks built on criminal law, judicial decisions, professional regulation, or parliamentary processes that have not yet matured into final legislation.

Switzerland and a Europe in Motion - Germany, Italy, France, and the United Kingdom

Switzerland is distinctive because its framework focuses on assistance in suicide under conditions that include, among other things, the absence of selfish motives on the part of the person assisting. It is not a classic medical statute authorizing a physician to perform euthanasia. Specialized organizations play an important role, and the person carries out the final act. Switzerland thus maintains a relatively sharp distinction between supplying assistance and performing the life-ending act.

The Swiss model has also led to travel from other countries seeking assistance, because the framework does not uniformly impose a residency requirement like those used in some jurisdictions. The phrase "suicide tourism" is charged, but the phenomenon raises genuine questions of equality and oversight: may a state become a destination for people whose own countries prohibit assistance, and how should capacity and voluntariness be assessed when the clinical relationship is brief?

Germany has experienced complex constitutional debate over prohibitions on organized assistance in suicide. Constitutional case law emphasized dimensions of self-determination, while the legislature continues to grapple with regulation. The German example shows that a constitutional judgment recognizing an underlying liberty does not immediately create a medical service. Between constitutional principle and practical pathway lie legislation, regulation, and professional controversy.

Italy has proceeded mainly through case law recognizing narrow circumstances in which assistance in suicide may not be punishable, while political disagreement continues. The model is not equivalent to the Netherlands. It shows how a court may create a limited exception where the legislature has not completed a comprehensive regime. For lawyers, the distinction between non-criminality under defined conditions and an entitlement to a service is essential.

France reached a parliamentary turning point in July 2026 when the National Assembly adopted at final reading a proposal to create a right to assistance in dying. As of August 14, 2026, however, the arrangement should not be described as a law already in force: after the final vote on July 15 the text was referred for review by the Constitutional Council, and the constitutional process had not yet been completed. This is a clear example of why a book documenting changing law must state the date of verification precisely.

At the same time, France strengthened its palliative-care and support framework in 2026 through Law No. 2026-404 of May 26, 2026. The separation between the two legislative tracks matters: expansion of palliative care can proceed even while the question of assistance in dying remains constitutionally and politically contested.

In the United Kingdom, the Terminally Ill Adults (End of Life) Bill from the 2024-2026 session did not complete its passage through the House of Lords and fell at the end of the session. On June 17, 2026, a new bill was introduced in the House of Commons for the 2026-2027 session; its text was published on July 16, and second reading was scheduled for September 11, 2026. Thus, as of August 14, 2026, the United Kingdom still had no general law permitting assisted dying under that bill, and the measure should be described as pending legislation.

These countries also illustrate the influence of human-rights courts and European legal frameworks. There is nevertheless no single European rule compelling every state to legalize euthanasia. National discretion remains broad, and states balance life, privacy, autonomy, and protection of vulnerable people in different ways.

For Israel, a "Europe in motion" may be more instructive than jurisdictions whose regimes are already settled. It shows how change occurs: a judgment, a committee, a bill, constitutional review, a pilot, and implementation. Any future reopening of the Israeli debate would require a choice not only about the result but also about the institutional route.

The European chapter therefore ends without a simple axis from conservative to liberal. Switzerland permits assistance in a manner unlike the Netherlands; Germany protects self-determination while still debating regulation; France stands between parliamentary adoption and constitutional review; and the United Kingdom remains in legislative debate. From here the comparison moves to Canada, whose broader MAID system has become one of the central international points of controversy.

Chapter 3

North America - Canada and the United States: Two Different Pathways to Medically Assisted Dying

Canada built its MAID pathway following constitutional litigation and then federal legislation that developed in stages. The model permits medical assistance in dying for people who meet statutory conditions and includes both practitioner-administered and, in certain structures, self-administered forms. The use of one term for two modes of performance is itself a reminder that MAID should not automatically be translated as "assisted suicide" alone.

Canadian legislation has, over time, distinguished between people whose natural death is reasonably foreseeable and those who do not fall within that pathway, with different safeguards. The development demonstrates how a law can expand beyond the classic terminally ill patient. The more remote natural death becomes, the more sharply the system must ask whether suffering, disability, and chronic illness can justify an irreversible pathway and what safeguards are required.

One particularly sensitive issue is mental illness as the sole underlying medical condition. As of August 14, 2026, eligibility where mental illness is the sole underlying medical condition remains excluded until March 17, 2027. The date matters because professional and public debate is continuing. Canada should not be described as already operating that pathway in full.

Canadian debate over disability is intense. Disability-rights organizations have argued that a person may obtain a pathway to death more quickly than housing, personal assistance, or treatment. Supporters respond that denying MAID to a competent person solely because of disability is paternalistic and discriminatory. The dispute illustrates that autonomy and equality can point in opposite directions.

The system requires professional assessments and, in some circumstances, enhanced waiting or safeguarding requirements. The important question is not merely how many checks exist, but what they examine: voluntariness, knowledge of alternatives, medical condition, and suffering. A formal mechanism can appear strong while remaining weak if alternatives are not genuinely accessible. The quality of health and social services is therefore part of any evaluation of the regime.

Canada also raises questions of access in remote areas and among Indigenous populations. A nationwide legal service can be experienced differently across provinces and communities. Culture, a history of harm within health systems, and mistrust require particular care. A formally universal right should not be assumed to be experienced identically by every population.

With respect to conscience, professionals and institutions face varying duties of referral and transfer depending on province and profession. The issue highlights the difference between ordinary health services and an act that a professional may regard as contrary to personal or professional identity. Any solution has to address patient access while protecting conscience to the extent recognized by law.

Canada publishes MAID data that allow monitoring of numbers, diagnoses, and characteristics. Growth in numbers, however, does not by itself prove either success or a slippery slope. Increases can reflect awareness, wider eligibility, demographic change, or improved access. Trends must be interpreted against legal and population changes.

For Israel, Canada is a test case of what happens when the debate moves beyond terminal illness and focuses on irreversible suffering and autonomy. It is also a methodological warning: a reform that appears narrow at the outset may change through legislation and case law, so any proposed change should consider in advance how future boundaries will be determined and who will have authority to alter them.

Canada is a federal system, but the United States presents an even more fragmented mosaic. There is no uniform national pathway; states that permit medical aid in dying tend to emphasize terminal illness, self-administration, and residency or other connection to the state in different ways.

United States - A Federation of Models, Not One Law

The United States neither "permits" nor "prohibits" assisted dying as a single national unit. Federal law leaves substantial space to the states, so the map changes over time. Oregon pioneered the Death with Dignity Act, and other states adopted similar pathways or variations. A common feature in many is terminal illness with a limited prognosis, a request by a competent adult, and self-administration of medication.

The self-administration requirement distinguishes these pathways from jurisdictions where a physician can perform the final act. It is intended to preserve final control in the patient's hands and distance the physician from direct killing. It also creates an equality problem: a person may satisfy eligibility criteria but lose the physical ability to swallow or administer the medication. States address this boundary in different ways.

Oregon developed a process involving requests, waiting periods, and confirmation of diagnosis that became a model for other states. Changes have occurred over time, including adjustments to some residency requirements. Comparison among state statutes requires current verification because details change. An old list of "legal states" is not reliable.

Washington, California, Vermont, Colorado, New Jersey, New Mexico, Hawaii, Maine, New York, and other frameworks reflect different developments. New York deserves particular note in this edition: its Medical Aid in Dying law took effect on August 5, 2026, only days before the manuscript date. The example shows how the legal map can change within weeks and why future printings require updated verification.

In many American pathways, terminal illness is defined by a prognosis of approximately six months. The criterion ties assistance to approaching natural death and narrows eligibility compared with Canada. Its weakness is prognostic imprecision and variation among diseases. A person with ALS may lose the physical capacity for self-administration before meeting the prognostic threshold, creating a difficult mismatch.

Insurance and private health care add a distinct dimension. Critics worry that insurers or health systems could favor a less expensive option; supporters emphasize safeguards and the patient's control. Trust requires a clear separation between coverage decisions and presentation of assisted dying. Any suggestion that financing influences the choice can damage legitimacy.

The physician's role varies by state, but typically involves confirming criteria and prescribing medication rather than performing the final act. This affects professional identity and conscientious objection. One physician may see the role as providing an option rather than killing, while another may reject the moral distinction. The law uses a practical boundary that allows some pluralism.

State data can be used to examine who uses the pathway, where death occurs, and what reasons people report. Loss of autonomy or control may appear alongside pain. This is a reminder that requests are not always responses to a symptom that can be measured. Policy must also address existential and functional concerns.

The United States also demonstrates the power of ballot initiatives and state legislation. Change can come directly through public voting and local political processes rather than only through courts. Campaign language, local data, and political context therefore matter greatly. Neighboring states can reach different outcomes on the same question.

For Israel, the American approach offers one example of a narrow pathway based on self-administration and terminal illness, but it is not a model that can simply be copied. Insurance arrangements, federalism, litigation culture, and attitudes toward medication and lethal means differ. The comparative value lies in seeing how design restrictions shape the population that becomes eligible. From North America, the book moves to a broader map in which South America, Australia, New Zealand, Asia, and Africa offer very different routes to end-of-life law.

Chapter 4

South America - Colombia, Ecuador, Uruguay, and Other Models

South America has in recent years become an unusual legal laboratory in end-of-life law. Contrary to the assumption that change concerning euthanasia always moves from the legislature to the health system, constitutional courts have led change in some countries, while legislatures have created explicit frameworks in others. Comparing Colombia, Ecuador, and Uruguay is especially valuable because they have reached partly similar outcomes through different institutions, and each has built a distinct structure of eligibility, oversight, and medical responsibility.

Colombia - From Constitutional Case Law to Regulation of the Service

Colombia is one of the clearest examples of a right to die with dignity developing over years through constitutional litigation. The starting point was Judgment C-239 of 1997, after which the doctrine expanded. In Judgment C-233 of 2021, the Constitutional Court removed the requirement that the person requesting euthanasia necessarily be terminally ill and focused instead on consent, a serious and incurable illness or injury, and intense physical or psychological suffering inconsistent with the person's conception of a dignified life. The center of gravity shifted from "how much time remains" toward a combination of severity, suffering, and autonomy.

The Colombian development is not limited to euthanasia. Judgment C-164 of 2022 also addressed asistencia médica al suicidio - medical assistance in suicide - and established a constitutional framework in which blanket criminalization of medical assistance can infringe fundamental rights when defined conditions are satisfied. The distinction is important: in euthanasia the physician performs the act that causes death; in physician-assisted suicide the person performs the final act after receiving medical assistance. For lawyers, the fact that both can be connected to the idea of a dignified death does not erase differences in liability, professional role, and oversight.

Colombian case law also illustrates the gap between recognition of a right and practical access. Later judgments addressed patients who encountered delays, restrictive interpretations, or system barriers. On April 29, 2026, the Colombian Ministry of Health issued Resolution 813, an updated regulatory framework addressing the right to die with dignity, euthanasia, and proportional adjustment of therapeutic effort. Institutionally, this represents a gradual shift from judicial recognition of a right to construction of a health service that must define who evaluates, who documents, who resolves disputes, and how patient wishes are preserved.

From a nursing perspective, such a model sharpens the need to recognize pressure, changes in wishes, or uncertainty about consent over time. A request that appears stable in one medical interview may sound different during a night shift, after a change in pain, or following a family encounter. That does not mean the nurse "approves" the request; the role is to bring relevant information to the team and ensure that the formal process remains connected to the patient's lived clinical reality.

Ecuador - Constitutional Judgment and a Developing Implementation Process

In Ecuador, the turning point was Judgment 67-23-IN/24 of February 5, 2024. The Constitutional Court established a framework under which, when the conditions defined in the judgment are met, a physician performing euthanasia at the request of a person suffering because of a serious and irreversible illness or injury would not incur criminal liability. The judgment relied on dignity, autonomy, and a life of dignity, but did not stop at an abstract principle; it required the authorities to advance implementation arrangements.

The Ministry of Health issued administrative regulation in April 2024 intended to make the judgment operational. The legislative process was not completed immediately, and in 2026 the Court and institutions were still following progress. The case teaches an important constitutional lesson: when a court opens an exception to criminal law, the health system still needs procedures, forms, designated authorities, appeal mechanisms, and professional guidance. A constitutional right that is not translated into a safe workflow can remain uneven among institutions.

Ecuador also has comparative significance for Israel. Both systems place strong weight on human dignity, but their normative starting points differ: the Israeli framework expressly maintains a boundary prohibiting an act intended to cause death, while Ecuadorian constitutional case law opened a route to active intervention under defined conditions. The comparison asks not only "who permits" but which institution made the decision and what happens when legal change moves faster than clinical infrastructure.

Uruguay - Explicit Parliamentary Legislation

Uruguay presents a different route. Law 20.431, enacted on October 24, 2025 and published on November 5, 2025, created an explicit euthanasia regime. Regulations were adopted in April 2026 by Decree 76/026. The law requires, among other things, adulthood and mental capacity, an incurable and irreversible medical condition under the statutory requirements, and suffering that the person considers unbearable or severe and progressive deterioration in quality of life. The process rests on a personal request, medical-record documentation, the ability to withdraw the request, and institutional oversight.

Especially important is that the Uruguayan law does not treat the act as a private decision between physician and patient alone. It places obligations on health-service providers and creates a review commission. The model reflects the view that once the state permits a medical act intended to cause death, autonomy by itself is not enough; monitoring, reporting, oversight, and equitable access are required. For an Israeli book, this is a relatively new legal experiment whose implementation should be followed over time rather than used for premature conclusions.

Argentina, Chile, Brazil, and Mexico - Intermediate Pathways

Express authorization of euthanasia is not the only way to expand patient liberty. In Argentina, Law 26.742 strengthened the patient's right to refuse certain treatments and leave advance directives, while also providing that advance directives requesting euthanasia are invalid. Conceptually, this model is closer to Israel: it expands control over the limits of intervention without turning a request for a lethal act into a legal entitlement.

In Chile, Brazil, and Mexico, the discussion includes varying combinations of patient rights, palliative care, advance wishes, state or local legislation, and proposals for legal change. There is no value in treating the region as a single unit. Federal structures, the power of constitutional adjudication, Catholic traditions, availability of palliative care, and health-system inequality all shape the practical meaning of "choice."

The central lesson from South America is that the legal route matters almost as much as the outcome. Colombia shows how developing case law can create a right and require the health system to build a service; Ecuador shows the tension between a constitutional judgment and completion of legislation; Uruguay offers explicit parliamentary legislation; and Argentina illustrates expanded autonomy without authorization of active euthanasia. For Israel, the comparison asks not only whether to change the boundary, but which institution should decide, what safeguards must come first, and what oversight is needed afterward.

Protecting Minors and Persons With Disabilities

Colombian law demonstrates how expanding a right requires redesigning safeguards when minors or people who have difficulty expressing wishes are involved. A 2025 judgment addressed, among other things, the difficulty of substitute consent involving a minor with cognitive disability and severe suffering. No simple rule should be extracted from such a case. On the contrary, it shows that the question of who speaks for the person becomes more complex as the intervention becomes more irreversible. Safeguards should move beyond group labels such as "minor" or "person with a disability" to individualized examination of ability, wishes, preferences, suffering, available treatment, and the risk that another person's decision will replace the patient's voice.

Comparatively, this is also a test of equality. A person with disability should not automatically be treated as living a life of lesser value, but should not be denied autonomy merely because of a diagnosis. Holding both principles at once requires a process that separates external judgments of quality of life from the person's own experience and requires the team to offer treatment and support before concluding that suffering cannot be relieved.

Constitutional Law and Health Services

Developments in the region illustrate a problem repeated throughout this book: a court can strike down a prohibition or recognize a right, but it does not run a hospital ward. After judgment come budgets, assigned roles, response times, committees, staff training, and a reporting system. If these are not built, the practical availability of the right depends on place of residence and institution. In this sense, accessibility is part of the substance of the right, not merely an administrative matter.

The comparison also reminds us that palliative care and assisted dying should not be framed as competing pathways. In any serious model, clinicians must ask what was offered to the person, which symptoms were treated, whether psychological and social support were available, and whether the person understands that requesting assisted dying is not a condition for receiving care. The more a state expands the boundaries of autonomy, the greater its responsibility to ensure that the decision did not arise because alternatives were unavailable.

Key official sources: Corte Constitucional de Colombia, C-233/2021 and C-164/2022; Ministerio de Salud y Protección Social, Resolución 813 de 2026; Corte Constitucional del Ecuador, Sentencia 67-23-IN/24 and follow-up materials; Uruguay, Ley 20.431 and Decreto 76/026; Argentina, Ley 26.742.

Chapter 5

Australia and New Zealand - Regulation, Oversight, and Differences Within Similar Models

Australia and New Zealand offer a useful comparison of assisted dying within developed public health systems that speak a broadly similar legal language but are institutionally organized in different ways. In Australia, regulation was built state by state and territory by territory; in New Zealand, a single national framework was created. The comparison shows how the same principles - capacity, free will, advanced illness, oversight, and conscientious objection - can take different forms depending on the structure of government and the culture of the health system.

Australia - A Federation of Similar but Non-Identical Models

Victoria was the modern Australian pioneer and commenced its Voluntary Assisted Dying pathway in 2019. The other states followed, and on November 3, 2025, the Australian Capital Territory (ACT) also began operating its regime. As of August 2026, the Australian framework is no longer a single-state experiment but a network of regional schemes, each setting eligibility requirements, a request process, medical assessments, reporting requirements, and oversight mechanisms.

The similarities among the models should not obscure their differences. In New South Wales, for example, the person must have an advanced and progressive disease or medical condition expected to cause death within the period defined by the legislation, with a longer horizon for neurodegenerative disease. The process includes a first request, assessment by a coordinating practitioner, a second independent assessment, a written declaration, and a final request. The multiplicity of steps is designed to create distance between a momentary statement and an irreversible decision.

The ACT adds an interesting form of administrative review. The territory's Civil and Administrative Tribunal can review certain decisions concerning capacity, voluntariness, and compliance with residency requirements. Legally, this is an important mechanism: it separates medical assessment from the possibility of reviewing defined elements of the decision without turning every request into full-scale litigation.

Victoria itself illustrates that regulation is not a one-time event. Amendments to its legislation were passed in November 2025, but they are not scheduled to take effect until April 2027; until then, the existing regime continues to govern. This is a useful example of why a legal text must distinguish between an amendment that has been enacted and a rule that already binds clinicians today. It also shows that end-of-life policy requires reassessment after practical experience accumulates.

Oversight, Documentation, and the Role of the Clinical Team

Across the Australian models, oversight does not end with the question whether the person meets eligibility criteria. The process also requires documentation, independent assessments, reporting, medication management, and clearly defined professional roles. Clinically, this requires coordination among primary care, specialists, pharmacy, nursing, and palliative care. The availability of VAD does not cancel the duty to treat pain, breathlessness, anxiety, or family needs.

The ACT expressly emphasizes that exploring or using VAD should not impair access to palliative care and other services. Ethically, this is a key principle: assisted dying must not become a cheaper substitute for care. Free choice requires the alternative of continuing to live with good treatment to be real rather than theoretical.

Nurses also have a distinct role. They may be the first to hear a request, notice that a person has changed his or her mind, detect signs of pressure, or observe that the clinical condition has changed. In a system that regulates VAD, professional boundaries must be clear: what may be explained, what requires referral, who assesses capacity, who may handle the medication, and what must be documented. Such clarity protects both the patient and the professional.

New Zealand - A National Framework, a Referendum, and Ongoing Monitoring

In New Zealand, the End of Life Choice Act 2019 came into force on November 7, 2021 after approval in a referendum. It allows a person who meets the statutory criteria to request medication to end his or her life. The national framework defines eligibility and safeguards, including age, citizenship or permanent-residency status, terminal illness with a life expectancy of less than six months, irreversible decline in physical capability, and capacity to make the decision.

The advantage of a national model is relative uniformity, but oversight remains necessary. The Registrar for assisted dying examines compliance with the process, receives reports, and handles complaints, while the End-of-Life Review Committee reviews reports concerning deaths. The Registrar's annual report published in July 2026 makes it possible to assess the service not merely at the level of legislation but at the level of implementation - essential for academic analysis, because a statute that looks sound on paper may still fail in accessibility or oversight.

The Act underwent its first statutory review in 2024. At the same time, attention was also given to how the service fits Maori communities and broader cultural obligations. This offers an important lesson for Israel: an end-of-life system should be culturally responsive, but cultural responsiveness must not replace the individual's wishes. The goal is to allow whanau or family to participate when the person wants that participation, not to assume that the group decides on the person's behalf.

Australia and New Zealand show that assisted-dying policy does not end on the day legislation comes into force. Authorization is followed by a long period of staff training, oversight, data collection, procedural amendment, management of conscientious objection, and monitoring of access. If Israel ever considers changing the limits of its law, this is the central lesson from the region: the normative decision is the beginning of planning, not the end.

Eligibility Is More Than a Diagnosis

In the Australian models, a serious disease alone is not enough. Assessment combines disease course, expected death, suffering, capacity, and voluntariness. A physician is therefore not merely asked to "confirm a diagnosis" but to make a clinical-legal judgment. One person may be gravely ill but fall outside the temporal criteria; another may satisfy the disease criteria but raise concerns about external pressure or ability to understand the process. Separating the components of eligibility prevents diagnosis from becoming a shortcut.

Differences among Australian jurisdictions also create a natural field for research. When two public health systems are similar but differ in waiting periods, residency requirements, method of administration, or obligations placed on institutions, it becomes possible to examine whether those differences affect access, delay, refusal, or safety. This is an advantage of federalism: variation allows learning, although its disadvantage is that a person may face different options on opposite sides of an internal border.

Conscientious Objection and Access

One practical challenge is how to respect a professional who is unwilling to participate while preventing institutional objection from erasing a right granted by law. Australian models regulate, in different ways, duties concerning information, referral, and institutional conduct. Ethically, no solution is cost-free: compelling a physician may impair professional integrity, while complete obstruction may make a legal right depend on the personal beliefs of the first clinician the patient happens to meet.

The problem is especially acute in rural and underserved areas. If authorized practitioners are scarce, distances are large, or appropriate pharmacy services are limited, a pathway designed for a metropolitan area may be nearly inaccessible in a remote community. Quality measures should therefore include not only case numbers but waiting times, travel distance, rates of incomplete referrals, and the availability of palliative care alongside VAD.

Data as a Mechanism of Accountability

A major strength of Australia and New Zealand is the accumulation of reports, reviews, and legislative evaluations. Such data permit debate to move from slogans to questions that can actually be studied: who applies, how many requests do not complete the process, how long people wait, which diseases are most common, and what role palliative care plays. In an academic book, it is important to separate a statistic describing use from a normative conclusion: an increase in the number of cases may reflect improved access, cultural change, or expansion of a system; by itself, it proves neither success nor failure.

Key official sources: Victoria Department of Health, Voluntary Assisted Dying; NSW Health, eligibility and process; ACT Voluntary Assisted Dying Act 2024 and Regulation 2025; New Zealand Ministry of Health, End of Life Choice Act framework and Registrar Annual Report 2026. 21

21. Victoria Department of Health, Voluntary Assisted Dying; amendments passed 18 November 2025, effective from April 2027; NSW Health, Voluntary Assisted Dying; ACT Voluntary Assisted Dying Act 2024 and Regulation 2025; New Zealand Ministry of Health, End of Life Choice Act framework and Registrar Annual Report 2026.

Chapter 6

India - The Right to Die with Dignity Without Permitting Active Euthanasia

India provides one of the most important comparisons with Israel because it recognizes a right to die with dignity and permits withholding or withdrawal of life-sustaining treatment, while not turning active euthanasia into a lawful medical service. Much of the development has occurred through the Supreme Court, showing how constitutional discourse about dignity and autonomy can expand control over the limits of treatment without necessarily adopting the Dutch model.

Common Cause - Autonomy, Advance Directives, and Withdrawal of Treatment

In Common Cause in 2018, the Supreme Court held that the right to life under Article 21 of the Constitution includes, in end-of-life circumstances, a right to die with dignity. The judgment recognized the right of a person with capacity to refuse life-sustaining treatment, the possibility of making an Advance Medical Directive, and a procedure for withholding or withdrawing treatment when the person lacks capacity, subject to procedural safeguards. At the same time, the Court emphasized that withdrawal of treatment does not eliminate palliative care and medical support.

The first problem with the model was its complexity. A mechanism designed to protect a person can make a right inaccessible if it requires too many approvals or procedures that do not fit clinical reality. In 2023, the Supreme Court simplified parts of the framework. The change illustrates a broader principle: procedural safeguards should reduce risk, but when they become too burdensome they create risk of their own - prolonging treatment against the person's wishes simply because the pathway cannot be completed in time.

Harish Rana, 2026 - Artificial Nutrition as Medical Treatment

On March 11, 2026, the Supreme Court issued Harish Rana v. Union of India, 2026 INSC 222, deepening the framework. Rana involved a man who had remained for years in a persistent vegetative state after severe brain injury and was fed through a PEG tube. The Court had to consider whether Clinically Assisted Nutrition and Hydration - nutrition and hydration supplied by medical means - constitutes "medical treatment" that can be withdrawn under end-of-life law, and what the patient's best-interests standard requires when he lacks capacity to express a wish.

The Court held that tube feeding can constitute medical treatment and that saying a person is "not connected to a ventilator" is not sufficient to remove the case from the framework. This rejected the idea that only an obvious mechanical device counts as life-sustaining treatment. The decision is particularly important in modern medicine: life support can be provided by tubes, pumps, medication, and continuing nursing processes, not only by a single machine that is switched on or off.

From a nursing perspective, PEG feeding is not an abstract legal concept. It requires care of the insertion site, assessment of tolerance, prevention of obstruction, management of aspiration risk, administration of medications, hygiene, and monitoring. When a court classifies artificial feeding as medical treatment, it is in effect recognizing the entire professional process that sustains it. A decision to withdraw it must therefore be translated into a clinical plan addressing mouth care, comfort, secretions, perceived thirst, family support, and symptom control.

Harish Rana also sharpened the best-interests test. Where there is no clear advance directive, the question is not what the family "wants" for itself, but what serves the individual in light of condition, prognosis, treatment burden, expected benefit, and identifiable values. The case illustrates why end-of-life law is not merely consent law: decisions sometimes have to be made for a person who cannot consent, and then process and evidence become the person's protection.

Law, Inequality, and Palliative Care

India requires comparative research to look beyond case law. A vast and unequal health system creates a gap between a constitutional right and practical ability to use it. The Ministry of Health operates the National Programme for Palliative Care, intended to integrate palliative services at district level, develop training, and strengthen community and home care. The existence of a program does not guarantee uniform availability, but it underscores that a right to refuse treatment must exist alongside the possibility of receiving treatment for pain and suffering.

Religion and culture add further depth. Hindu, Muslim, Christian, Sikh, and Buddhist traditions coexist, and families may play a central role in decision-making. There is therefore no single "Indian position." A legal system that recognizes autonomy should take family relationships and belief into account, but it should not assume that an individual necessarily wants what his or her community is presumed to want.

The lesson for Israel is significant. Both countries try to distinguish an act intended to cause death from withholding or withdrawing treatment. India, however, shows that categories evolve when a court confronts a specific technology - here, artificial nutrition - and interprets it according to the purpose and nature of treatment rather than simply its physical form. Israel may face similar disputes as home technologies, pumps, and support systems become more complex.

A Medical Process Instead of a Single Decision-Maker

One feature of the Indian framework is the use of medical boards and multi-stage assessment when the patient cannot express a wish. The rationale resembles protective mechanisms in Israel: the more irreversible the decision and the weaker the evidence of the person's wishes, the less appropriate it is to leave the decision to one individual. A committee, however, is not a guarantee of quality. It is useful only if members receive complete information, distinguish prognosis from value judgment, and document reasoning rather than merely the result.

Harish Rana also demonstrates the importance of distinguishing the cause of death from the treatment decision. Withdrawal of medically assisted nutrition is not described as administering a lethal substance; the law asks whether continued intervention is beneficial and whether the underlying disease or injury may be allowed to take its course. Philosophers may dispute the distinction, but legally it determines which rules apply and which authorization is required.

Advance Directives in a Family-Centered Society

An Advance Medical Directive may look like an individualistic instrument, but in India it often operates within a family that is deeply involved in care. This is both a strength and a risk. Family members may preserve knowledge about the person's values and protect those values when communication is lost; they may also exert pressure or find it difficult to accept a document that conflicts with their own wishes. A well-prepared directive should therefore be accompanied, where the person wishes, by prior discussion with relatives to reduce the gap between a written instruction and a future crisis.

Nursing again forms a crucial implementation link. A decision to stop a particular treatment is not the end of care: it requires a detailed plan for comfort, mouth and skin care, prevention of distress, medication adjustment, and support for relatives. This reinforces the distinction on which the book repeatedly relies - stopping one intervention is not stopping professional responsibility.

India as a Mirror for Israel

The similarity between the two countries is not that their laws are identical, but that both attempt to maintain a moral and legal line between "not prolonging" and "causing death." The mechanisms differ: in Israel the distinctions were designed in a detailed dedicated statute; in India much of the framework developed through constitutional adjudication. The comparison permits examination of the clarity offered by legislation against the flexibility of case law that can adapt general principles to new technologies.

Key official sources: Supreme Court of India, Common Cause v. Union of India (2018); Harish Rana v. Union of India, 2026 INSC 222, 11 March 2026; Directorate General of Health Services, National Programme for Palliative Care. 22

22. Supreme Court of India, Common Cause v Union of India (2018); Harish Rana v Union of India, 2026 INSC 222, 11 March 2026; Directorate General of Health Services, National Programme for Palliative Care.

Chapter 7

East Asia - South Korea, Taiwan, Singapore, and Japan

East Asia is important to comparative study because it disproves any simple equation between autonomy and permission for euthanasia. South Korea, Taiwan, and Singapore have built detailed systems for advance planning, refusal of treatment, and decisions about life-sustaining care without adopting a model identical to the Netherlands. Japan adds a system in which much of the regulation rests on professional guidance, case law, and a distinctive decision-making culture. The family's role is especially prominent in the region, making it useful for examining forms of autonomy that are not exclusively individualistic.

South Korea - National Registration and an Institutional Process

South Korea's Act on Decisions on Life-Sustaining Treatment for Patients in Hospice and Palliative Care or at the End of Life created a regulated system of Advance Directives and Life-Sustaining Treatment Plans. A person aged nineteen or older may complete an advance directive after receiving an explanation at a registration institution recognized by the Ministry of Health. The document is entered into a national system and can be amended or revoked. The structure gives importance not only to wishes but also to verification, explanation, and the ability to retrieve the document when it is needed.

Organizationally, the Korean model also includes institutional ethics committees and a national information-management mechanism. This is an important point for Israel: a legal document is useful only if a team in an emergency department or ward can know that it exists, verify its validity, and interpret it in relation to the present clinical condition. Digital registration is not merely administrative; it is part of the ability to translate earlier autonomy into a clinical decision.

Taiwan - The Patient's Right to Autonomy

Taiwan's Patient Right to Autonomy Act provides a broad framework for advance planning and treatment decisions in defined circumstances. After a planning and counseling process, it allows a person to state in advance his or her wishes concerning life-sustaining treatment and artificial nutrition and hydration when specified clinical conditions arise. The framework is especially interesting because it does not stop with the question whether someone is "terminally ill"; it seeks to connect advance planning with a range of circumstances in which autonomy may be lost in the future.

The Taiwanese model also shows why Advance Care Planning is more than a form. An advance decision about feeding, ventilation, or another treatment requires understanding how the person views dependence, consciousness, suffering, and meaning in life. When the conversation occurs before a crisis, clinicians can explore values rather than merely check boxes. This is particularly relevant to possible reform in Israel, where complex forms and low awareness can leave formal rights largely unused.

Singapore - An Advance Medical Directive Without Euthanasia

In Singapore, an Advance Medical Directive is a legal document that a person over the age of twenty-one can execute to direct that extraordinary life-sustaining treatment not be used when he or she is terminally ill and unconscious or otherwise unable to communicate, under the conditions set by law. The Ministry of Health emphasizes that the decision is voluntary and that coercing a person to make an AMD is an offense. The regime is also expressly distinguished from euthanasia and assisted suicide.

Singapore has in recent years broadened public discussion through Advance Care Planning and digital tools for documenting preferences. The distinction between an AMD and ACP matters: the former is a relatively focused legal instrument; the latter is a broader process for discussing treatment goals, values, and the people the patient wishes to involve. From a nursing perspective, ACP can be particularly valuable because it supplies context where a form does not provide a binary answer.

Japan - When Regulation Is More Dispersed

Japan does not have a comprehensive national pathway for euthanasia or medically assisted dying comparable to permissive European models. End-of-life decisions rely more heavily on general medical law, professional guidance, case law, and institutional judgment. Families often receive considerable weight, but it would be wrong to infer that every Japanese patient prefers family decision-making. Individual preferences about communication, disclosure, and family involvement still have to be identified.

Relational Autonomy and Its Meaning for the Clinical Team

Comparison across East Asia shows that autonomy can be relational rather than isolated. Research on shared decision-making in contexts influenced by Confucian familism suggests that family can form part of a person's identity and decision-making process. The difference from paternalism is that the clinical team does not assume in advance that the family decides; it asks the person what role he or she wants the family to play.

In practice, the four systems emphasize the importance of locating prior wishes, culturally adapted explanation, and the danger of withholding information in the name of "protecting" the patient. Nurses and physicians need communication skills that allow them to ask not only what should be decided but how the person wants the decision to be made. East Asia therefore adds a dimension that a purely European comparison can miss: the right to choose includes the choice of whether to choose alone.

Israel can draw a practical lesson from this. In a multicultural society, advance-directive systems should not be built around one model of family involvement. A person can be allowed to define who receives information, who participates in discussion, who acts as proxy, and which values should guide that proxy. Law can thus preserve family involvement without permitting the family to erase the individual's voice.

Advance Planning as Public Policy

A feature shared by the three systems with explicit legislation is that advance planning is not treated as a purely private matter. Registration, counseling, recognized forms, and accessible information turn the person's wishes into part of health-system infrastructure. This matters because, in an emergency, there is little time to search for an unfamiliar document or interpret a sentence written without professional explanation. Advance planning works when it is connected to the record, the clinical team, and an implementation process.

The Korean model particularly demonstrates the advantage of a national registry. A document intended to operate only in the future is practically valid only if it can be found. Legally, this is a reminder that a right requires an information architecture. From a nursing perspective, access to information reduces the likelihood that relatives and clinicians will argue at the bedside while the patient's preference is already recorded somewhere no one can locate.

Taiwan adds another dimension: an advance process that connects clinical conditions to values. The more a document addresses states of consciousness, artificial nutrition, and life-sustaining treatment, the greater the need to explain what those terms mean. Legally, agreement to an unexplained term is not autonomy. The quality of counseling before the document is therefore almost as important as the signature itself.

Between Confidentiality, Truth, and Family Harmony

In systems where family is central, conflict may arise over disclosure of diagnosis. A family asking clinicians "not to tell" may be acting out of love, but concealment can prevent the person from planning care, saying goodbye, or preparing a directive. The professional response is to identify the patient's own information preferences in advance. A person may choose to have family receive information first; that is an autonomous choice and differs from the family appropriating the right for itself.

The regional discussion also shows that cultural difference is not an exemption from professional standards. Family pressure, delirium, depression, or misunderstanding of treatment can arise in every culture. Cultural sensitivity should improve assessment, not lower the threshold. Precisely where family is deeply involved, clinicians need to document who said what, what the patient wanted, and how contradictions between individual wishes and family expectations were resolved.

The Comparative Lesson

East Asia demonstrates that expanding autonomy does not necessarily lead in a straight line toward euthanasia. A system can create national registries, early counseling, recognition of treatment withdrawal, and structured family involvement while maintaining a prohibition on acts directly intended to cause death. This makes the region especially relevant to Israel, which may wish to strengthen implementation of patient wishes without necessarily abandoning the normative boundary in its existing law.

Key official sources: Republic of Korea, Act on Decisions on Life-Sustaining Treatment and National Agency for Management of Life-Sustaining Treatment; Taiwan, Patient Right to Autonomy Act; Singapore Ministry of Health, Advance Medical Directive. Supplementary research: Yang Y et al., Confucian Familism and Shared Decision Making in End-of-Life Care, 2022. 23

23. Republic of Korea, Act on Decisions on Life-Sustaining Treatment; Taiwan, Patient Right to Autonomy Act; Singapore Ministry of Health, Advance Medical Directive; Yang Y et al. Confucian Familism and Shared Decision Making in End-of-Life Care. 2022.

Chapter 8

Africa - Law, Palliative Care, and Health Justice

Africa changes the perspective of the debate. Much of the literature on assisted dying comes from countries with developed palliative-care systems, making it easy to assume that every person chooses among several medically available alternatives. In countries and regions where access to oncology, hospice, home care, and analgesia is severely limited, autonomy looks different. Before asking whether the state should provide a medical route to death, one must ask whether it provides a reasonable way to live through the end of life without unnecessary pain.

South Africa - Constitutional Law and the Criminal-Law Boundary

South Africa is the continent's principal legal test case. In 2015, the High Court in Stransham-Ford granted an individual application that opened a path to assisted dying in the circumstances of that case. In 2016, however, the Supreme Court of Appeal reversed the decision. Among other things, it emphasized procedural limitations and the need not to create a broad change in criminal law through an individual case that had lost much of its practical significance after the applicant's death. The result is that the case remains an important focus of debate but is not a simple basis for claiming that assisted death became a generally lawful service in South Africa.

The significance of the case lies in more than the outcome. South Africa's Constitution gives central place to dignity, liberty, and bodily rights, while criminal law protects life. The tension resembles constitutional disputes elsewhere, but the judicial decision highlights an institutional question: should a court create an exception, or should the legislature build criteria, oversight, and rules for conscientious objection after public deliberation?

The history of legal-reform discussion in South Africa also shows that the question is not new. Committees and studies have considered treatment limitation, advance directives, and assisted dying over many years. The fact that lengthy debate has not produced a national Dutch-style model is not simply "lack of development"; it shows that non-change is also a legal choice with institutional and social reasons behind it.

Other Countries - Caution Against Overgeneralization

In the examples examined, including Kenya and Nigeria, criminal law does not present medically assisted dying as a regulated legal service comparable to Canada or Australia. That does not mean every end-of-life decision is prohibited. Systems that strongly protect life still face separate questions about refusal of treatment, medically futile treatment, determination of death, palliative care, and professional guidance. Academic comparison must avoid the error in which "no euthanasia" becomes "no end-of-life law."

Palliative Justice - Without a Real Alternative, Choice Is Incomplete

The World Health Organization estimates that tens of millions of people worldwide need palliative care each year and that only a minority receive it. The burden falls heavily on low- and middle-income countries; among children, almost half of those needing palliative care live in Africa. This changes the normative debate: if pain, breathlessness, and psychosocial support are not treated, a request to die may be influenced by a deprivation that could have been reduced.

Access to morphine is a concrete example. Overly restrictive regulation, procurement difficulties, fear of addiction, and lack of training can leave people without basic pain relief. WHO emphasizes the need for balance: preventing nonmedical use must not block essential medicines. Uganda's experience, where oral-morphine supply models were developed through cooperation between government and hospice services, shows that progress can occur independently of any debate about euthanasia.

From a nursing perspective, palliative justice is also a workforce issue. Where specialist physicians are scarce, nurses, community health workers, and volunteers may play central roles in recognizing pain, educating families, administering medication, and monitoring patients at home. End-of-life policy must therefore ask who can actually deliver care in practice, not only who is formally authorized on paper.

Religion, Community, and Family

Africa has no single culture and no single religion. Christianity, Islam, local traditions, and different family structures coexist, and in some contexts family and community are deeply involved in decisions. Here too, the collective must not become a substitute for consent. The clinical team's task is to ask the patient whom he or she wants involved and to distinguish community support from pressure that narrows freedom.

Africa's contribution to this book is not the question "which country will be first to permit assisted dying?" but the prior condition it brings into focus: autonomy requires infrastructure. A society that speaks about a right to choose the timing of death while failing to provide pain control, a supportive home, basic equipment, or family assistance offers a defective choice. Conversely, service gaps are not in themselves an eternal answer against legal change; they are a moral demand that any change be assessed together with health justice.

For Israel, where palliative care exists but is not always equally accessible, the lesson is direct. Debate about the boundaries of the Dying Patient Law should include not only formal rights but distribution of services, specialist availability, home care, and nursing education. The African comparison returns the book from constitutional theory to the practical capacity of a health system to deliver what it promises.

Health Infrastructure as a Condition for Meaningful Choice

The palliative gap raises a question of priorities. It does not mean autonomous rights must "wait" until a health system is perfect; no health system is perfect. But when basic analgesics, home services, or trained teams are lacking, the state should ask whether what appears to be an individual choice is being shaped by systemic failure. That is the difference between respecting a wish and normalizing deprivation.

WHO emphasizes that palliative care includes physical, psychological, social, and spiritual dimensions and should be integrated into primary and community care. In regions where hospitals are far away, home-based models are not merely a preference but may be the only way to reach people. Training nurses and community health workers is therefore part of the infrastructure of end-of-life rights.

Morphine as a Test of Balanced Regulation

Difficulty in accessing opioids shows how a law intended to protect can cause harm. Regulation of controlled medicines is essential, but licensing, procurement, and storage rules that do not fit real conditions can prevent appropriate care. Current WHO guidance seeks a balance between safety and availability. The same way of thinking is relevant to assisted-dying policy:

protection should not become blind obstruction, and autonomy should not become unregulated permission.

Health justice also includes people who do not have cancer. Heart failure, lung disease, HIV, neurological disease, renal failure, and frailty in old age can all cause severe suffering. A system that identifies palliative care only with oncology misses large groups. At population level, expanding these services may change how people understand their options near the end of life.

Knowledge and Data

A major difficulty in comparative research on Africa is the lack of uniform data. Absence of data does not prove absence of practice, but neither does it justify filling gaps with assumptions. This chapter therefore uses a strict approach: where no clear legal framework or implementation data can be verified, it does not rank the country but describes what can be established and the policy questions that remain open.

For the same reason, Africa should not be depicted as an "early stage" on a path toward a European model. The aim is not to assume that every country will move in one direction, but to understand how dignity, religion, family, resources, and criminal law shape local answers. Good comparison respects the possibility that societies may arrive at different balances even after considering the same evidence.

Chapter 9

The Global Matrix - Not "Permitted or Prohibited," but a Continuum of Regulatory Models

After surveying different jurisdictions, it becomes clear that there are not merely two categories. At least five regulatory models can be identified: a broad prohibition alongside a right to refuse treatment; regulation of withholding and withdrawal through advance directives; assistance in suicide only; euthanasia and assisted dying in terminal illness; and broader models that do not require death to be near. 24

Meaningful comparison requires a fixed series of questions. Must there be terminal illness? Is an incurable disease enough? Who performs the final act? Are minors included? What is the status of mental illness? Are advance directives recognized? How many professionals are required? Is there a waiting period? Does the system review each case before or after the act? What is the status of conscientious objection? Is the service publicly funded?

Israel occupies a distinctive middle position. It broadly recognizes advance planning and withholding treatment under defined conditions, yet prohibits a direct act intended to cause death and limits withdrawal of continuous treatment. It is more permissive than systems without effective advance-directive mechanisms, but it remains far from models that permit euthanasia.

There is no objective hierarchy of "advanced" and "outdated." Each model assigns different weight to values and risks. Academically, the important question is not which country is more "enlightened," but what price each system is prepared to pay in order to protect the value it prioritizes.

A useful comparative matrix begins with the threshold question: who is eligible. Some countries require terminal illness and short life expectancy; others require a serious and irreversible medical condition and suffering; still others permit no active assistance at all. The very first row already shows that the word "permitted" conceals very different populations.

The second question is who performs the act. In the Netherlands and Belgium, a physician may perform euthanasia under specified conditions; in many American jurisdictions, the individual must self-administer; Canada provides different pathways; and Switzerland's structure focuses on assistance rather than physician-administered euthanasia. This difference affects people with physical limitations and shapes the physician's professional role.

The third question concerns capacity and wishes. Almost every permissive model requires a voluntary request, but rules concerning advance directives, dementia, and minors differ. The Netherlands allows some role for advance directives in a broader context; many systems require capacity at the time of the act. Inclusion of minors is rare and tightly limited.

The fourth question is prognosis. Many American models tie eligibility to approximately six months, whereas the Netherlands and Belgium are not built solely around such a time window. Canada has extended eligibility beyond reasonably foreseeable death in some circumstances. Prognostic criteria therefore shape both which diseases qualify and when access becomes possible.

The fifth question is suffering. Must suffering be physical, psychological, or both? Must it be "unbearable"? Who evaluates it? Must alternatives merely be offered or actually tried? A subjective term needs procedure if it is not to become an unlimited gate.

The sixth question is oversight. The Netherlands relies on regional retrospective review; Spain includes a pre-authorization evaluation body; other jurisdictions require reporting to a health authority. Review after the event is faster but depends on accurate reporting, while prior authorization can prevent error but may cause delay. No model is perfect; each chooses among risks.

The seventh question is conscience. May a physician refuse? Must he or she refer? What happens when an institution objects? A patient's legal right can be meaningless without providers, yet forcing a professional to participate can impair freedom of conscience and professional culture. Every country constructs a different balance.

The eighth question is palliation. Does the law require alternatives to be offered? Are services genuinely available? Is there parallel investment in palliative care? Serious comparison cannot stop with statutory wording. Real access changes how free a request actually is.

The ninth question is data and transparency. Public reports make research possible, but researchers must understand what is being counted. A statistic on euthanasia is not necessarily a statistic on MAID, and a report on prescriptions is not necessarily a count of deaths. A matrix must therefore define the variable as well as display the number.

Israel appears in this matrix as a system that recognizes refusal, advance directives, and withholding of certain treatments for a dying patient, while prohibiting active euthanasia and assisted suicide. The comparison does not place Israel "behind" or "ahead." It shows where its law draws the boundary and which value that boundary protects.

The matrix also shows that a country need not import an entire foreign model. Israel can learn about registries, reminders, oversight, communication, and palliation without changing the prohibition on euthanasia. If it ever considers assisted dying, however, it will have to define eligibility explicitly rather than rely on a broad label.

Summary Matrix: Five Regulatory Patterns

The matrix is an analytical tool, not a substitute for the country chapters. Every system contains exceptions, threshold requirements, and changes over time; each row should therefore be read alongside the relevant jurisdictional chapter and the date on which the law was checked.

From here, the discussion can move from comparative doctrine to normative debate. After seeing what countries do, the next question is why they do it and which arguments are strongest for and against. The following discussion does not seek to "win" the debate, but to distinguish value arguments, empirical claims, and institutional concerns.

24. Emanuel EJ, Onwuteaka-Philipsen BD, Urwin JW, Cohen J. Attitudes and Practices of Euthanasia and Physician-Assisted Suicide in the United States, Canada, and Europe. JAMA. 2016;316(1):79-90.

Chapter 10

China and Thailand - Advance Directives and Digital End-of-Life Planning

After India and Japan have been discussed in their dedicated chapters, two further models are worth examining primarily for implementation: Shenzhen in China and Thailand. Neither provides a pathway comparable to the Dutch model of active euthanasia. Their comparative significance lies instead in how an advance wish moves from an abstract document to information that can be located and acted upon within the health system.

Shenzhen - Local Recognition of Directives in a Vast System

In Shenzhen, a local arrangement that took effect in 2023 recognizes patients' advance wishes at the end of life concerning interventions such as intubation, resuscitation, and life-support measures. The comparative significance is not that China adopted a uniform nationwide right, but that a major city can function as a regulatory laboratory within a much larger system. For other countries, this shows how change may begin with documentation and implementation even before national resolution of every end-of-life issue.

Thailand - From a Legal Right to an e-Living Will

Thailand's framework recognizes a declaration in which a person asks not to receive services intended only to prolong life in the terminal phase, and in recent years it has added a digital dimension through an e-Living Will. The important innovation is not simply the ability to complete a form online, but the idea that advance wishes can form part of an information infrastructure: a document that can be updated, verified, and found when the person can no longer explain it.

The Systemic Lesson: A Document That Cannot Be Found in Time Does Not Implement Autonomy

Both models emphasize that digitization is not merely scanning a paper form. A reliable system must identify the valid version, connect it securely to the patient's identity, display critical instructions to clinicians quickly, and permit updating and revocation. It should also avoid alert overload, because a warning that appears at every encounter can become background noise that staff learn to ignore.

For Israel, the comparison is useful precisely because it does not require moving the criminal-law boundary. Israel can learn how to make existing directives more available during hospitalization, how to design reminders and validity renewal, and how to connect prior wishes with the medical record without assuming that a document alone replaces discussion. The lesson is about infrastructure and implementation, not expansion of eligibility for assisted dying.

Chapter 11

Muslim Countries - Sanctity of Life, Medically Futile Treatment, and the Boundary Against Euthanasia

Saudi Arabia - Prohibition of Euthanasia Alongside Recognition of Medically Futile Treatment

Ethical rules governing health professionals in Saudi Arabia place a clear prohibition on participation in euthanasia or assisted suicide, including administration of a substance with the purpose of causing death. The normative boundary is therefore explicit.

At the same time, those rules recognize a patient's refusal of therapeutic interventions after appropriate information has been provided and, in incurable situations, acknowledge that there is no obligation to begin - and in some circumstances it may be permissible to discontinue - advanced measures from which no benefit is expected, subject to professional assessment and specialist decision-making. The duty to treat pain and other symptoms continues.

The Saudi model matters because it shows that the distinction between "killing" and "not prolonging medically futile treatment" is not unique to Jewish tradition or Israeli law. It also exists in modern Muslim medical ethics. This creates room for shared discussion in multireligious societies: agreement about limits of treatment does not require agreement about euthanasia.

United Arab Emirates - An Explicit Legislative Prohibition

Federal law in the United Arab Emirates provides that a patient's life may not be ended, even at the patient's request or the request of a guardian. This is a direct formulation that places the boundary in medical-liability law rather than leaving it solely to an ethical code.

The UAE example illustrates a model of normative certainty: clinicians do not have to guess whether a patient's request authorizes an act directly intended to cause death. Yet certainty about the prohibition does not by itself answer questions about advance care, withdrawal of medically futile interventions, or relief of suffering. The quality of end-of-life policy therefore cannot be measured only by whether euthanasia is lawful.

Egypt, Saudi Arabia, and the United Arab Emirates together offer an important conclusion for Israel. A relatively religious and conservative model can reject active assistance in dying while still needing to distinguish preservation of life from prolongation of a futile dying process. Where that distinction is translated clearly into clinical practice, suffering can be reduced without changing the criminal-law boundary.

Chapter 12

Ten Practical Lessons for Israel

1. Separate Two Questions That Israeli Debate Often Blends Together

The first question is how to make the existing law work better. The second is whether to move the boundary and permit active assistance in dying. There is no reason to make improvement of the first depend on resolution of the second.

Japan and Thailand do not need to legalize euthanasia in order to invest in care planning, repeated conversations, and digital tools. Israel too can improve advance directives, expand access to palliative care, and create faster decision pathways without changing a single provision in the prohibition on active euthanasia.

2. Reconsider the Six-Month Rule

Comparison shows at least three alternatives. Canada uses whether death is reasonably foreseeable to determine the level of safeguards. Colombia removed terminal illness as an absolute condition for its pathway. The Australian Capital Territory requires an advanced and progressive condition expected to cause death but does not impose a fixed number of months.

This does not mean Israel should abolish the six-month limit. The more modest conclusion is that the current boundary is not the only possible way to protect patients. Israel could consider an additional route for irreversible neurodegenerative diseases, especially where the person has capacity or where a clear advance directive exists, without adopting a model of euthanasia.

3. Treat Prognosis as an Assessment With Uncertainty, Not a Binary Fact

Oregon demonstrates clearly that a person may satisfy a six-month prognosis at the time of assessment and in fact live longer. In Israel, physicians, committees, and courts should not treat prognosis as though it were a scientifically fixed expiration date. The basis of the estimate and its uncertainty should be documented, rather than allowing a small difference between two statistical assessments to determine whether a person has fundamental end-of-life rights.

4. Choose Deliberately Between Prior Review and Retrospective Oversight

The Netherlands and Belgium demonstrate the advantages of systematic review after the event; Spain and Ecuador place greater weight on review before action. There is no single correct answer for every type of decision.

Israel can classify decisions. Relatively routine decisions not to start treatment in accordance with a valid directive should not require a burdensome committee process; a genuine dispute over capacity, wishes, or withdrawal of complex treatment may justify prior review. Retrospective sample-based or systematic review can then be used to learn whether the mechanism is functioning properly.

5. Establish Binding Time Frames

Data from Spain demonstrate that time is part of the right. In Israel too, a person whose life is measured in weeks cannot meaningfully rely on a bureaucratic answer that arrives after death.

Legislation or regulations should provide both an ordinary route and an urgent route, with short and clear deadlines for committee decisions, second opinions, and appeals. Safeguards need not disappear, but they must operate at a pace compatible with end-of-life medicine.

6. Turn Advance Directives Into an Active Digital System

Thailand and Shenzhen offer a practical direction. Israel already has a national registry, but it could be transformed from a document repository into an active clinical system: digital signature, guided completion, linkage with health plans and hospitals, alerts on admission, the ability for the patient to update preferences, and automatic reminders before expiration.

In such a system, the team should not need to ask relatives whether "there might be a document at home." The existence of a directive should be part of the core information available to the physician, much like a medication allergy or current medication list.

7. Ensure Palliative Care Before Choice Becomes a Debate About Death

India, Switzerland, Thailand, and other jurisdictions emphasize in different ways that an end-of-life treatment decision does not eliminate the duty of care. Stopping ventilation, dialysis, or artificial feeding should not create a therapeutic void.

Israel should consider a clear standard: before major decisions not to prolong life, and certainly before any future discussion of assisted dying, patients should be offered appropriate palliative assessment, treatment of pain and breathlessness, psychological support, and assistance for the family. Palliative care should not become a "test" that invalidates the patient's wishes; its purpose is to ensure that the choice is not being driven by treatable pain or by absence of any alternative.

8. Protect Professional Conscience Without Allowing Patient Abandonment

The Netherlands does not compel a particular physician to perform euthanasia. Uruguay recognizes conscientious objection but requires continuity of access. The principle can be applied in Israel regardless of whether legalization is considered.

A physician or nurse should not be forced to perform an act that deeply violates conscience, except where an emergency creates an independent duty to treat. At the same time, a public institution should not leave a patient without information or a clear point of contact. The law should distinguish personal conscience from institutional obstruction.

9. Publish Annual Data Rather Than Rely on Anecdotes

Belgium, Spain, Oregon, and other jurisdictions regularly publish data on implementation. Israel needs the same data culture even under its existing law.

How many people were formally defined as dying patients? In how many cases was an advance directive available? How many matters were referred to committees and how long did they take? In which diseases did disputes arise? How often was a document invalid or inaccessible? How many patients received palliative consultation?

Without data, it is impossible to know whether a problem is rare or systemic. Public debate also becomes more vulnerable to extreme stories that may not represent the overall picture.

10. Build Periodic Review Into the Law

Austria approved amendments in July 2026, including a more flexible renewal mechanism scheduled to enter into force on February 1, 2027; Victoria has already adopted changes due to commence in 2027; and the ACT is examining an issue that became apparent almost immediately after implementation. By contrast, the core of Israel's framework was set in 2005, in a medical and technological world very different from that of 2026.

A sensitive law should not change with every change of government. Precisely for that reason, a structured review mechanism is desirable: for example, every five years a professional-public committee could examine implementation data, new technologies, diseases that remain insufficiently addressed, access to palliative care, and public attitudes, and submit a public report to the Knesset.

Periodic review does not require amendment. It requires the state to know why it is leaving the law as it stands.

Chapter 13

What Must Not Be Learned Automatically from Comparative Law

Comparative law can be an extremely useful tool, but it can also become a dangerous shortcut. The fact that a particular European country permits an act does not prove that the same rule fits Israel. Conversely, the fact that a religious country prohibits it does not prove that prohibition is necessarily the right answer for Israel.

Law operates within culture. Trust in physicians, family structure, access to health services, economic inequality, the place of religion, center-periphery relations, the quality of care for older people and persons with disabilities, and the availability of home care all affect the practical meaning of the same legal rule.

For example, a right to choose death has a different meaning in a system where every person has real access to home hospice, pain treatment, and a caregiver than in a system where a family faces financial collapse to keep a person at home. Likewise, a prohibition on euthanasia looks different when a patient can be confident that unwanted invasive treatments will not be forced on him or her than when the prohibition is accompanied by difficulty refusing intervention.

Israel should therefore not begin with the question, "Which country should we copy?" It should begin with local questions: where does the current law fail; which patients fall outside the framework; are advance directives accessible; is palliative care available equitably; what does the public understand; and what level of protection is needed in a society where family plays a central role in medical decisions?

Only after those questions are answered should a tool from another country be selected.

Chapter 14

Autonomy and Whether a "Right to Die" Exists at All

The Argument From Autonomy: "My Life, My Decision"

Autonomy is one of the strongest concepts in modern medicine. It does not mean that the patient becomes his or her own physician; it means that medical decisions concerning the person's body cannot be examined only through the question of what professionals are capable of doing. They also require attention to wishes, values, worldview, and the price the person is or is not willing to pay for prolongation of life. 25

In the end-of-life context, the autonomy argument becomes particularly powerful. When cure is no longer possible, treatment may mean prolonging life at the cost of dependence, pain, functional decline, or a way of living that conflicts with the person's conception of dignity. Those who support broader choice argue that it is precisely then that the person should not become an object of decisions made by others. If the person has capacity, understands the condition and alternatives, and expresses a consistent wish, that wish should carry decisive weight at least in relation to refusal of treatment.

The phrase "my life, my decision," however, does not end the debate. In medicine, almost no important decision occurs in a completely private sphere. It involves professionals, relatives, institutions, and law. As the request moves from refusal of a medical intervention toward a demand for an act whose direct purpose is to cause death, a second question is added to the patient's liberty: does one person's freedom create an obligation for another person to perform an act that the latter regards as immoral or outside the proper role of medicine?

Autonomy is therefore not a magic word. It is a powerful principle operating alongside others: prevention of harm, protection of vulnerable persons, medical professionalism, equality, and the design of public policy that looks not only at private choice but also at the conditions under which the choice was formed.

Supporters of assisted dying argue that the distinction is insufficient. If a competent person may refuse ventilation and die, why should another person who is not dependent on a machine but suffers just as severely be unable to receive assistance? The difference in outcome may be medically accidental.

In their view, genuine autonomy should focus on suffering and control rather than on which technology happens to keep the person alive.

Opponents respond that autonomy is not a right to every service. A person cannot demand removal of a healthy organ or a dangerous drug without indication merely because it is his or her body. Medicine and the state may define some acts as outside legitimate medical practice. The question therefore becomes one about the role of the physician, not only ownership of the body.

Autonomy also depends on alternatives. Choosing death when there is no access to symptom relief, housing, or support may be voluntary in a narrow sense but heavily shaped by deprivation. Supporters argue that a person should not lose a choice because the state has failed; opponents fear that the state may offer death instead of repairing the failure. Both positions require social policy, not merely a capacity test.

A further problem is change of mind. People may ask to die at one point and later adapt. For this reason, different regimes require repeated requests, waiting periods, or opportunities to withdraw. Such safeguards treat autonomy as a process rather than a moment. Yet a waiting period that is too long can make the right inaccessible to a person whose condition is deteriorating.

Autonomy also includes the right to choose life. In a society where assisted dying is lawful, an older or disabled person must not feel that he or she is expected to "consider" it. The very presentation of the option can be experienced as pressure depending on who raises it and in what setting. Communication rules therefore matter: a right to receive information is not a duty to justify continuing to live.

The autonomy argument is strongest where the person has capacity, is consistent and informed, and is free from pressure. The hard cases begin when one of those conditions weakens: depression, financial dependence, family messaging, or uncertain prognosis. Legislation is not written only for ideal cases and therefore needs mechanisms for recognizing the boundaries.

Philosophically, autonomy can be understood not as ownership but as authorship of one's life story. On that view, a person seeks an ending consistent with the values by which life has been lived. The argument can support advance directives, choice of place of death, and refusal of treatment without necessarily supporting euthanasia. A person who values autonomy is not logically committed to every model of assisted dying.

In Israeli law, autonomy carries significant weight in relation to treatment but stops at the boundary of an act intentionally designed to cause death. That boundary can be criticized, but it should be described accurately. The debate is not between a system that respects autonomy and one that does not; it concerns the scope of autonomy.

The autonomy argument supplies the foundation for discussion, but turning it into a legal claim requires identifying against whom the right is asserted and what it obliges that person or institution to do. The rest of this chapter therefore asks whether it is meaningful to speak of a "right to die" at all and, if so, in what sense.

Relational Autonomy, Not Legal Isolation

Medical autonomy protects people against decisions being made over their heads. It does not assume that human beings exist outside relationships. Serious illness affects spouses, children, and caregivers, and sometimes the person explicitly wants decision-making to be shared. Law that respects autonomy should also allow a person to choose to involve others, provided involvement does not become coercion.

The difficult task is identifying pressure. A request that follows family comments about financial burden or accusations of "selfishness" requires different scrutiny from a consistent request made within a supportive relationship. There is no perfect test of authenticity, but private discussion with the patient, time, and capacity assessment can reveal improper influence.

Autonomy also includes the right to change one's mind. A decision about treatment or an end-of-life pathway is not an irrevocable contract. A system that makes withdrawal from a request difficult undermines the very value it claims to protect.

The autonomy argument becomes specifically legal only when we ask what follows from it. The freedom to choose is not necessarily identical to a right to demand an act from another person, so freedom from unwanted treatment must be distinguished from a claim to active assistance in dying.

Does a "Right to Die" Exist at All?

The phrase "right to die" attracts public attention because it sounds clear and decisive. Legally, it is far more complex. Rights can be negative, protecting a person against coercion or interference, or positive, imposing a duty on the state or another person to act. This distinction fundamentally changes end-of-life analysis.

The right of a competent person to refuse treatment is a classic negative right: the body belongs to the person, and the system may not impose a medical intervention merely because it might prolong life. A demand for lethal medication, or for clinicians to perform an act intended to cause death, is different. It does not simply ask the state to leave the person alone; it asks the state to establish a professional pathway that makes death possible.

For this reason, courts and legislatures around the world have reached different results even when all recognize dignity and liberty. A state may recognize refusal of treatment without recognizing a right to assistance in dying. It may allow assistance in self-administration but not physician-performed euthanasia. It may permit both under strict conditions. These outcomes are not necessarily contradictory; they reflect different conceptions of how far society is prepared to impose a duty on others.

The phrase "right to die" can therefore obscure more than it reveals. Precise analysis should ask which right is claimed, against whom, what act it requires, and which safeguards are needed to ensure that it is not exercised under pressure, error, temporary despair, or lack of alternative care.

The right to refuse treatment largely arises from bodily integrity. If a competent person says, "Do not touch me," treatment without consent requires exceptional justification. Death may be a consequence of refusal, but the state is not necessarily "granting a right to death." It is recognizing a limit on power over the body. This formulation matters because it separates the content of the right from its possible result.

A right to assistance requires identification of a service provider. If no physician is willing to participate, must the state employ someone who will? Must insurance pay? Must a religious institution allow it? Once something is called a right, duties follow. Legislatures may therefore choose a model of criminal-law protection without defining a positive health service, or alternatively integrate the service into the health system.

Constitutional rights such as dignity, privacy, and liberty may support the claim, but they can be limited. The state may argue that restrictions protect vulnerable persons, trust in medicine, and life itself. A court must then ask whether the prohibition is proportionate and whether less restrictive alternatives exist. The answer depends on the local constitutional structure.

A right also raises equality questions. If only a person who can travel abroad or discontinue a machine can control the circumstances of death, others may claim discrimination. Conversely, assisting a person with disability because he or she cannot perform the act independently may raise concern that the state is helping precisely a vulnerable group to die. Equality does not point in only one direction.

The right to life is not necessarily a duty to remain alive. In human-rights law, protection of life requires the state to prevent arbitrary killing and build safeguards, but whether it requires forced treatment of a competent person is a different question. Distinguishing right from duty prevents slogans from doing the work of legal analysis.

There is also a conceptual question whether "death" can be the object of a right at all. Rights generally protect interests held by living persons; after death there is no rights-holder in the same sense. Supporters answer that the right concerns choice of timing and manner while the individual is alive. The linguistic dispute reflects a deeper disagreement over what law is protecting.

Different jurisdictions use alternative formulations: right to die with dignity, aid in dying, assisted dying, death with dignity. Each frames the phenomenon differently. "Suicide" emphasizes self-action; "assisted dying" is more medicalized; "death with dignity" is value-laden. Academic legal analysis has to move from the label to the operative rule.

In Israel, as of the time of writing, there is no legal right to receive euthanasia or assistance in suicide. There are substantial rights concerning refusal of treatment and advance directives within the applicable legal frameworks. Use of the phrase "right to die" without clarification can therefore create a misleading impression.

The discussion of rights naturally leads to why people seek them. One powerful argument is compassion in the face of suffering. But "unbearable suffering" is complex: it may involve pain, loss of control, fear, or loss of meaning. The next chapter examines this concept without assuming that all suffering is medical in the same way.

Constitutional courts around the world have reached different results because constitutions assign different weight to dignity, life, privacy, and liberty. Even when a court recognizes end-of-life autonomy, it may leave the legislature broad room to design safeguards. Constitutional rights are not always ready-made answers; often they define the boundaries of the question.

From a medical perspective, the language of rights changes behavior. If a patient believes he or she has a "right" to a particular act, a physician's refusal may be understood as a violation rather than as professional judgment. Precise language is therefore important: who is entitled to request, who is entitled to receive, and when may a professional refuse? Linguistic accuracy is part of fairness.

25. Washington v Glucksberg, 521 U.S. 702 (1997); Vacco v Quill, 521 U.S. 793 (1997); Pretty v United Kingdom, App. No. 2346/02, European Court of Human Rights (2002).

Chapter 15

The "Slippery Slope" - Argument or Reality?

The slippery-slope argument appears in almost every debate about assisted dying, but it becomes useful only when we define what, exactly, is supposed to "slip." There are at least three distinct claims. The first is normative: once a principle is accepted for one group, pressure will arise to extend it to another. The second is empirical: the number of cases or the categories of eligibility will in fact expand. The third is institutional: safeguards will weaken over time. Mixing the three creates a debate in which each side appears to prove something different.

What the Data Show - and What They Do Not Show

In the Netherlands, 10,341 cases of euthanasia and assisted suicide were reported in 2025 under the statutory framework, representing 5.97 percent of all deaths; in seven cases the regional review committees found that not all due-care requirements had been met. In Belgium, 4,486 cases were reported in 2025, approximately 4 percent of all deaths. In Canada, 16,499 people received medical assistance in dying in 2024; 95.6 percent belonged to the pathway in which natural death was reasonably foreseeable, and 4.4 percent to the pathway in which it was not reasonably foreseeable.

In Oregon, 637 prescriptions were reported in 2025 and 400 deaths occurred after ingestion of the medication, with the latter figure subject to later revision.

These figures prove that use of the legal frameworks is not static and that there are substantial differences among jurisdictions. By themselves, however, they do not prove erosion. Growth may reflect population aging, increased awareness, an explicit legislative amendment, removal of a geographic barrier, or better reporting. To speak meaningfully about a slippery slope, one must identify in advance the change regarded as the risk and then ask whether it occurred because of expansive interpretation, legislative change, or failure of safeguards.

Belgium illustrates why precision matters. One case involving a minor was reported in 2025, and only seven such cases had been reported in total since the law was extended to minors in 2014. The legal possibility itself is a significant normative expansion; the very small number of cases is a separate empirical fact. An opponent of the expansion may argue that opening the category is itself the problem, while a supporter may point to the rarity of its use. Both propositions can be true at the same time because they answer different questions.

Canada illustrates another kind of expansion. A pathway exists for persons whose natural death is not reasonably foreseeable, yet in 2024 it represented 4.4 percent of cases. That figure allows the scale of use to be monitored, but it does not by itself answer whether the eligibility criteria are normatively appropriate. This is precisely why public reports should include not merely a total number, but also information about diagnoses, age, access to palliative services, social supports, the circumstances of the request, and cases that were declined or withdrawn.

Oregon demonstrates the need to distinguish an entry criterion from the eventual outcome. The law requires a prognosis of terminal illness, yet 24 of the 400 participants who died in 2025 lived for more than six months after receiving the prescription. This is not, by itself, a breach: prognosis is an assessment made at a particular point in time, not a guaranteed date. From a policy perspective, the figure is a reminder that any threshold expressed in months must acknowledge medical uncertainty.

How to Test Whether Safeguards Are Eroding

An empirical assessment should track at least four measures. The first is change in the eligibility criteria themselves. The second is the proportion of cases that do not fit the traditional interpretation of the statute. The third is the activity of oversight mechanisms - how many files were found noncompliant, referred for additional review, or led to changes in guidance. The fourth is the availability of alternatives such as palliative care and support for persons with disabilities. Without all four, it is difficult to determine whether a system is expanding through deliberate democratic choice or through uncontrolled erosion.

The opposite direction should also be examined. A system that is so afraid of exceptions that it makes refusal of treatment difficult, delays appropriate sedation, or fails to honor valid directives can create a "slippery slope of overtreatment." A sound evaluation therefore asks not only whether there were more assisted-dying cases, but also whether people received treatments they did not want and whether end-of-life safeguards operated in time.

For Israel, the principal lesson is methodological. If the boundaries of the law are ever reconsidered, the state should determine in advance what data will be collected, who will publish them, which changes require new legislation, and which body may interpret the conditions. That converts the slippery-slope argument from a claim based on fear or confidence into a mechanism of scrutiny: define the risk, measure it, and require the state to explain every material change.

Chapter 16

Are Acts and Omissions Morally Different?

The Question Cannot Be Resolved by Outcome Alone

One of the deepest controversies in end-of-life care is whether there is a moral difference between performing an act that brings about an outcome and refraining from an act that would have prevented it. The comparison becomes especially sharp when the outcome is death. Is administering a substance with the purpose of causing death fundamentally different from not starting a treatment, or from withdrawing a treatment after which disease causes death? The fact that the person dies in both situations does not decide the issue, because morality and law examine not only outcome but also intention, duty, causation, authority, and the identity of the actor.

The argument for a distinction emphasizes that the physician did not create the disease. When a patient refuses a medical intervention, the team ceases to place the patient's body at the disposal of technology and the disease continues its course. By contrast, when the intervention itself is intended to cause death, death becomes the goal of the professional act. From this perspective, the difference is not merely between physical "action" and "inaction," but between different purposes of professional conduct.

Critics point to situations in which the distinction appears artificial. If a treatment is keeping a person alive and withdrawing it is expected to lead to death within minutes, it is difficult to say that the team simply "did nothing." Moreover, a device designed to operate automatically makes continuation the default and stopping it an act, whereas a device requiring reactivation every hour would transform the same clinical decision into a series of omissions. If technology determines who appears active and who appears passive, it is reasonable to ask how much moral weight should rest on that technical structure.

Withholding Versus Withdrawing - Ethical Symmetry and Emotional Difference

Many medical ethics codes tend to regard withholding and withdrawing treatment as two forms of the same decision when treatment is unwanted or no longer advances the patient's goals. The American Medical Association Code of Medical Ethics, for example, states that there is no ethical difference between withholding and withdrawing life-sustaining treatment, while acknowledging that the emotional experience may differ. The logic is that if a patient may refuse treatment before it begins, agreement to a trial should not imprison the patient in that treatment after it becomes clear that it is no longer appropriate.

At the same time, professional and human emotions have institutional significance. A nurse who turns off a pump or a physician who discontinues support may experience responsibility differently from someone who never initiated the treatment. There is no reason to dismiss that experience as "irrational"; it affects moral distress, clinicians' willingness to act, and trust. But the intensity of the feeling should not, by itself, become the source of a right or a prohibition. Regulation should acknowledge conscience and emotional experience without making the patient's rights dependent on the psychology of whichever professional happens to be present.

Intention, Foreseeability, and the Cause of Death

Intention is not the same as knowledge that a result is foreseeable. A physician may know that stopping treatment will allow death to occur sooner while intending to respect a refusal or to discontinue treatment that no longer benefits the patient. Knowing that death is expected does not necessarily make death the purpose. Conversely, a subjective declaration of benevolent intent is not enough to justify every action; law and medicine also examine dose, professional standard, documentation, alternatives, and context.

Causation is also complex. When ventilation is withdrawn from a patient whose disease does not permit independent breathing, the withdrawal decision clearly affects the timing of death. There is no need to deny that fact in order to distinguish it from injecting a lethal substance. The accurate analysis is that two causal factors operate together: the disease created the dependence, and the clinical decision removed support. The moral question is what that influence means when the decision rests on the patient's wishes, treatment goals, and the governing law.

Why Law Still Needs Lines

Philosophy can leave a question unresolved; a clinical team cannot. At the bedside, a decision must be capable of implementation and documentation. Legal systems therefore use practical distinctions even where philosophical agreement is incomplete. Israel gave this distinction a distinctive form through the categories of continuous and cyclical treatment. The relevant question is not whether philosophy has "proved" the statute, but whether the chosen line achieves its purpose consistently and avoids unreasonable results.

Two criticisms should be separated. One argues that the Israeli line is difficult to implement or overly dependent on the technical structure of the treatment; that is a criticism of the regulatory instrument. The other argues that there is no moral distinction at all between causing death and allowing death; that is a far broader claim. One can accept the first criticism without accepting the second. Reform could alter the rules governing withdrawal of support without legalizing active euthanasia.

The Case of a Time-Limited Treatment Trial

A time-limited trial offers a practical means of reducing the tension. Rather than present a family with a choice between "do not start" and an open-ended commitment, the parties agree in advance to a defined period of treatment, set clinical goals, and establish a point for reassessment. If the goals are not achieved, returning to the discussion is not a retreat but part of the original agreement. This approach does not solve every legal question in Israel, but it reduces the error in which merely starting treatment acquires the moral status of a promise to continue it forever.

Ultimately, the distinction between acts and omissions is neither a myth that can be erased in a sentence nor an absolute truth that resolves every case. It is one of several layers of responsibility. A careful analysis of an end-of-life decision should ask what duty existed, who made the decision, what its purpose was, what medically caused the death, what the patient wanted, and what alternatives were available. Only the full picture permits a distinction among respecting a medical boundary, withdrawing treatment, and performing an act whose purpose is death.

An Omission Is Not Neutral When a Duty to Act Exists

Everyday language sometimes describes an omission as a situation in which "we did nothing," but in law and in the caring professions, inaction can carry full responsibility. A physician on call who fails to give antibiotics for a reversible infection despite a clear indication and a patient's wish to be treated does not become less responsible merely because no harmful substance was injected; the omission itself may breach a duty. The act-omission distinction therefore cannot operate alone. One must ask whether a duty to act existed and what that duty required at the relevant moment.

At the end of life, the content of the duty changes with the clinical situation and the goals of care. Sometimes the duty is to begin treatment, sometimes to offer a limited trial, and sometimes to refrain from an intervention the patient has rejected. The same physical "non-action" can constitute negligence, respect for autonomy, or sound clinical judgment. This is why legal analysis must begin with the relationship of duties rather than with the physical form of the conduct.

Moral Responsibility and Legal Responsibility Do Not Fully Overlap

A person may believe that there is morally no difference between two routes to the same outcome and nevertheless accept that law may distinguish between them in order to create clear boundaries, protect trust, and facilitate oversight. Conversely, law may classify two acts differently even when a clinician experiences them as morally equivalent. This tension is not a defect; it reflects different functions. Morality asks what ought to be done, while law must also ask what rule can be formulated, proved, and enforced.

Accordingly, debate about changing Israeli law should be cautious about the claim that "if there is no moral difference, there can be no legal difference." Even a critic of the present distinction must propose an alternative institutional mechanism: who is authorized to act, under what conditions, how the decision is documented, what role a second opinion plays, and how the system prevents a shift from withdrawal of treatment to an act intended to cause death. Without institutional answers, a philosophical argument is not yet a policy.

Chapter 17

Is the Physician's Role Always to Save Lives?

Medicine That Cannot Cure Must Still Care

The statement "the physician's role is to save lives" expresses an important truth, but it does not exhaust the profession. Physicians treat incurable diseases, chronic conditions, and people whose lives are approaching their end every day. They prevent disease, rehabilitate, relieve pain and breathlessness, explain, accompany, and help patients make decisions. If saving life were medicine's only goal, every death would be a professional failure and palliative care would be understood as surrender. Modern medicine rejects both conclusions.

The World Medical Association's Declaration of Venice on End-of-Life Medical Care emphasizes that the end of life is part of a person's life and that palliative care, autonomy, shared decision-making, and physical, psychological, social, and spiritual needs all deserve attention. This conception does not weaken the duty to rescue in an acute reversible condition; it places that duty within a wider system of goals. When an effective intervention can restore a person from a reversible state, the expectation to act is strong. When treatment no longer changes the disease and adds only burden, the professional question changes.

A Duty of Care Is Not a Duty to Use Technology

The existence of a device or procedure does not, by itself, create an indication to use it. Mechanical ventilation, dialysis, surgery, and oncological treatment are tools; the question is what they can achieve for this particular person. Professional competence includes the ability to offer treatment when appropriate and the ability to say that treatment is not appropriate when it has no reasonable benefit in relation to the goal. A competent patient may refuse a medically reasonable treatment, but autonomy does not necessarily create a right to demand from every physician an intervention that has no medical basis.

The term "futile" requires caution because it can blur facts and values. A treatment may have virtually no chance of achieving a physiological goal - for example, resuscitation that is not expected to restore circulation - or it may achieve a biological goal while still failing to produce an outcome the patient regards as meaningful. The physician should say which goal is not achievable rather than replace that statement with a judgment about the value of the person's life. This preserves the distinction between judging a treatment and judging a person.

Truth, Hope, and the Courage to Recommend

Protecting hope does not require concealing prognosis. Sometimes the absence of an honest conversation causes a person to choose treatment inconsistent with his or her goals because the patient believes the probability of benefit is higher than the team believes it to be. The physician's role is not to place a menu of options on the table and say, "You decide." Expertise also includes a recommendation. A sound recommendation states the uncertainty, explains what treatment can and cannot accomplish, and connects the information to the values expressed by the patient.

Hope itself can change form. When cure is no longer possible, a person may hope for time at home, a day without pain, a conversation with a child, a period of lucidity, or the possibility of not being alone. A physician who recognizes multiple goals is not "taking away hope"; the physician is helping move hope from an unattainable objective to goals that remain possible. That transition is part of treatment, not a conversation that takes place after treatment has ended.

The Boundary the Profession Sets for Itself

The debate over euthanasia and medically assisted dying reaches the core of professional identity because it asks whether causing death can, under some conditions, become a medical means of relieving suffering. The World Medical Association continues to oppose euthanasia and physician-assisted suicide while distinguishing them from respecting a patient's right to refuse treatment. Jurisdictions that have chosen differently have built pathways defining eligibility, oversight, and conscientious objection. The variation itself shows that the controversy is not purely medical; it is normative and social.

Even in a society that permits assisted dying, the physician's conscience is not a marginal issue. Compelling a professional to perform an act regarded as contrary to professional identity may harm both the practitioner and trust in medicine. At the same time, personal conscience should not become the power to block information or abandon a patient. Systems therefore need clear pathways for transfer, consultation, and continuity of care. The balance between conscience and access is part of health-system design, not merely a private disagreement between two people.

Moral Distress and Responsibility Toward the Team

End-of-life care produces moral distress even without euthanasia. A clinician may feel that harm is being caused when aggressive treatment continues despite lack of benefit, or may feel guilt when treatment is stopped and death follows soon afterward. A system that expects professionals to carry this tension alone risks emotional numbing, avoidance of difficult conversations, and defensive medicine. Team discussions, support, ethics consultation, and a shared language of treatment goals are professional safety mechanisms.

The answer to whether the physician's role is always to save lives therefore depends on what "saving" means. Physicians are committed to life, but not to every act that prolongs a biological process. They are committed to the person: to trying to cure when cure is possible, to prolonging life when that is consistent with reasonable goals and the patient's wishes, and to relieving and accompanying when cure is no longer possible. Forgoing a particular treatment can be a medical decision; giving up on the person cannot be one.

Who Defines Professional Success at the End of Life?

Medical culture is also shaped by the measures through which it rewards itself. A department that measures success almost exclusively by survival, procedures, and discharge may experience every transition to comfort-focused care as failure. If it also measures symptom control, quality of communication, concordance with patient goals, and avoidance of nonbeneficial interventions, professional space emerges for goals other than cure.

This does not diminish the value of survival. It prevents one measure from driving the team against the overall clinical picture. Excellent intensive care should know how to save a person who can be saved, but also how to recognize when support no longer achieves an outcome the patient would accept. Excellent palliative care should relieve suffering without assuming that every prolongation of life is a burden. Success is defined in relation to the goal, not the identity of the department.

Training for a Complex Professional Identity

For medical students it is easier to learn a resuscitation algorithm than to learn how to tell a person that there is no further curative treatment. The first can be practiced technically; the second requires language, tolerance of uncertainty, and the ability to remain in the room when there is no solution. Education in end-of-life care should therefore begin early and should not be reserved for palliative subspecialists.

Simulation of prognostic conversations, joint learning with nurses and social workers, and discussion of cases in which treatment achieved a physiological effect without advancing the patient's goals can build a professional identity that does not oscillate between two extremes - "do everything" and "give up." A physician who understands relief and accompaniment as medical acts can make end-of-life decisions without experiencing them as abandonment of the profession's mission.

Shared Decision-Making Is Not the Transfer of Responsibility to the Patient

The transition from paternalism to autonomy has sometimes produced the opposite mistake: instead of the physician deciding alone, the clinician presents a list of options and transfers the full weight of the decision to a sick person. Genuine shared decision-making does not mean, "Here are the options; choose." It requires the physician to make a professional recommendation, explain why it is recommended, identify the patient's values, and revise the recommendation when those values support a different path.

At the end of life, the distinction is critical because the options are not symmetrical and the information is not simple. A patient may hear, "We can attempt resuscitation," and interpret that as a promise of a meaningful chance of returning to function, while the team merely means that the procedure is technically possible. Professional responsibility requires translating technical possibility into an expected outcome. Only then does the choice truly belong to the patient rather than to the wording of the question.

Some patients explicitly ask for a strong recommendation. They are not necessarily surrendering autonomy; they are using the physician's expertise as part of their own decision. A physician can say, "In light of what you have told me matters to you, I recommend that we not perform this intervention," while leaving room for questions and refusal. In that way, professional responsibility is preserved without returning to a model in which the patient's wishes are pushed aside.

Chapter 18

The Person Behind the Law - Identity, Dependence, Fear, and Changing Wishes

There Is No "Generic Patient"

End-of-life legislation must use categories: dying patient, competent person, proxy, life-prolonging treatment. At the bedside those categories dissolve back into a particular human being. Two people with the same diagnosis, prognosis, and level of function may choose entirely different paths. One may want every additional day because of an approaching family event, because life itself carries overriding value, or because the person is not ready to let go. Another may regard another hospitalization as a price he or she no longer wishes to pay. The quality of a system is measured by its ability not to turn either person into the norm against which the other is judged.

The difference is not limited to treatment preference. A person reaches the end of life with a biography, beliefs, profession, relationships, habits, and a sense of identity. Serious illness narrows the range of choices, which can make the choices that remain unusually important: when to get up, who may enter the room, whether to remain lucid even at the price of some pain, whether to go home, what to tell the children, and when to tell them. A law that protects autonomy only at the moment a form is signed misses a substantial part of the autonomy a patient experiences in everyday life.

The Changing Body and the Experience of Dependence

Loss of independence can be as difficult as a physical symptom. A person accustomed to showering alone, using the bathroom without assistance, or managing the day independently may become dependent on others for intimate activities. Law cannot eliminate dependence, but professional care can address it: ask permission before touching, cover the body, explain what is about to be done, offer choice where choice exists, and avoid talking about the patient as though the patient were absent. These small acts give concrete meaning to human dignity.

Experience is not fixed. What a healthy person imagines as "a life I would never want" may feel different when the person actually lives with disability and discovers new sources of meaning. Conversely, a patient may discover that a treatment undertaken in the hope of recovery imposes a burden the patient is no longer willing to bear. Assessment of quality of life must therefore be cautious: it is not a score assigned by an expert from outside, but a combination of function, suffering, and the meaning the person gives to the condition.

When a Person Says, "I Don't Want to Be a Burden"

That sentence can sound like a clear position about continued life, yet it may contain very different concerns: fear of financial cost, guilt over a partner's exhaustion, lack of privacy, concern that children will miss work, or a sense that the system already regards the person as a burden. A response that rushes to say, "You are not a burden," may close the conversation. It is better to ask what, exactly, feels burdensome. Sometimes home assistance, benefits, social support, equipment, or respite for the caregiver can change the conditions - and with them, the meaning of the request.

The inquiry is not intended to persuade a person to choose life at any cost. It is intended to ensure that the decision is not the product of a remediable problem or, in reality, a request for help. This is an important distinction between respecting autonomy and being indifferent. A system that respects choice must also be willing to invest in the conditions that allow choice to be free.

Time, Fatigue, and the Way Information Is Delivered

A person near the end of life is often asked to receive complex information precisely when strength is diminishing. Pain, breathlessness, medication, fatigue, and anxiety can affect the ability to listen. Adapting communication does not mean reducing the amount or quality of information; it means changing the method: a shorter conversation, information in smaller segments, returning another day, simple written material, the presence of a person chosen by the patient, or an alternative communication aid. A person can be fully competent and still need better conditions in order to exercise that competence.

Time itself becomes a medical resource. A test that consumes an entire day in hospital may carry a substantial cost when only weeks remain. A medical intervention is not neutral merely because it is not especially dangerous; it consumes time, energy, and the ability to be elsewhere. At the end of life, the simple question "Will the result of this test change what we do?" may be more important than it would be when the person's horizon is long.

The Right to Know and the Right Not to Manage the End of Life Alone

Autonomy does not require a person to become the manager of his or her own death. Some patients want every detail and to make decisions themselves. Others want the physician to provide a clear recommendation. Still others want the family to participate centrally or even to carry part of the decision-making burden. When the choice of how to share decisions comes from the patient, it too is an expression of autonomy. A system that forces a person to decide alone in the name of freedom can become paternalistic in a new form.

Likewise, privacy does not disappear because family members are involved. A patient may want some information withheld from a particular relative or may ask to speak with the team alone. Illness does not abolish personal boundaries. Precisely when many people are speaking around and for the patient, it remains important to ask who should be in the room and what the patient wants them to know.

Fear, Hope, and Meaning

Fear of death is not always fear of pain. It may be fear of the unknown, loss of control, separation, disappearance, or concern for those who will remain. Some fears cannot be treated with medication. Conversation, spiritual, psychological or community support, and presence can be treatment in the deepest sense. There is no reason to assume that a religious person necessarily wants maximal treatment or that a secular person necessarily wants maximal control; meaning grows out of the individual's own world.

Hope also does not disappear when approaching death is acknowledged. A person may hope to be awake for a birthday, to hear music, to get home, or to finish a conversation. Recognizing these goals helps the team construct care whose success is not measured only in days. It also reminds everyone that the remaining time is still life, not merely waiting for death.

Changing Wishes Are Not a Failure of Planning

A treatment plan or an advance directive is intended to protect a person's wishes, not imprison them. A competent person may change his or her mind. The patient may accept a treatment previously refused or ask to stop a treatment that was undertaken in the hope of a different outcome. Change is not necessarily inconsistency; it can be a response to new information and to an experience that could not have been fully imagined in advance. The team should therefore return to the conversation when the situation changes rather than treat an old document as a substitute for the person standing before them.

This principle leads to the book's final substantive question: if dignity does not reside in one place, one form, or one decision, what makes the path toward death dignified? One element is the place in which a person receives care and dies - yet here too there is no single answer that fits everyone.

Legacy, Unfinished Business, and the Life That Remains

Near the end of life, people sometimes focus on what they will leave behind: a message to their children, a family story, an object, a photograph, reconciliation, or a practical matter long postponed. These needs are not "outside medicine" merely because they do not have a procedure code. Tests and hospitalizations can consume the time required for them; thoughtful planning can preserve that time. The team is not responsible for managing a person's legacy, but it can ask what still matters to complete and adapt decisions when possible.

This also changes the meaning of benefit. Another day in hospital for a test that will not alter treatment may have little value for a person who wants to spend that day at home. Conversely, a short treatment that allows someone to attend a family event may be highly valuable even if it does not change the long-term course of disease. As time grows short, goals that are not "medical" in the narrow sense become part of medical decision-making.

The Right to Ordinary Life Even During Terminal Illness

The end of life should not turn every moment into a farewell ritual. Some people want to speak about death; others want to watch a game, argue about the news, drink coffee, or sleep without another conversation about goals of care. A system that respects a person must also allow ordinary life. Excessive focus on illness can erase the life that remains just as completely as total denial of illness.

In practical terms, not every encounter should be made into a heavy decision point. Once a good plan has been built, the patient should be allowed simply to live within it. Planning is supposed to reduce repeated crises, not convert the end of life into an endless series of forms and conversations.

Intimacy, Touch, and Body Image

Advanced illness changes not only function but also the way a person experiences the body. A stoma, catheter, edema, wounds, weight loss, or the need for help with bathing can affect intimacy and identity. At the end of life, clinicians can become so focused on urgent symptoms that they miss the fact that the patient still wants to decide who sees the body, when the door is closed, and how care is delivered.

Touch is not self-evidently welcome. One person wants a hand held; another does not want to be touched. Some patients seek physical or sexual intimacy even during serious illness, and the system can make privacy possible rather than assume intimacy ends with a terminal diagnosis. Respect for the body is not an aesthetic issue; it is part of how a person continues to experience ownership of the self while many areas of control are being lost.

For nurses this point is especially professional. Bodily care occurs repeatedly throughout the day, so asking permission, giving a short explanation, and maintaining appropriate covering can shape the experience of dignity more powerfully than a general declaration of rights. Every action need not become a long conversation; consistent routine is precisely what creates the sense that the patient remains present in decisions concerning the body.

Chapter 19

Place of Death - Home, Hospice, and Hospital, and What "Death with Dignity" Means in Practice

Place of Death Is Not a Single Measure of Quality

In palliative-care discourse, death at home is sometimes presented as the preferred goal. Home has clear advantages: a familiar environment, privacy, greater control over visitors, and avoidance of some of the interventions and transfers of hospital care. Many studies indeed find that home is the preferred place of death for a large proportion of patients. Yet preference is not universal and may change. An umbrella review published in 2024 found that in the meta-analyses it included, roughly half of patients preferred to die at home, while substantial groups preferred hospice, a palliative institution, or hospital.

A high-quality system should therefore not be judged by the proportion of home deaths alone. It should be judged by its ability to identify a preference, offer genuine alternatives, and revise the plan when circumstances change. A person who wanted to die at home but chose transfer to hospice when breathlessness became severe did not "fail" the plan. The planning succeeded if it allowed the person to change direction without guilt and without chaos.

Home - Control and Closeness, but Dependence on Infrastructure

Home allows a person to remain in a familiar world: one's own bed, sounds, smells, belongings, and chosen people. Noise and testing can be reduced; the person can eat when desired and able, set the pace of the day, and preserve privacy. For someone who wants to avoid repeated hospitalizations, remaining at home can itself be a major treatment goal.

But a home does not become a hospice merely because it is a home. High-quality home care requires staff availability, medications, equipment, instruction, and a line to call when pain, secretions, agitation, or a change in breathing occurs. In Israel, the Ministry of Health states that home-hospice services are provided in the community as part of health-fund services. Formal entitlement matters, but the equality test is real availability: Is the service accessible in every region? Can medication be obtained at night? Will someone come when symptoms change? Can the primary caregiver bear the responsibility?

Recent reviews of home palliative care indicate the potential to reduce hospitalizations and increase the possibility of dying at home, but outcomes depend on the organization of the service and on family and system capacity. A home plan must therefore include a safety plan, not merely a preference: who calls whom, which medications are kept at home, when an ambulance should be called, which interventions are desired during an acute event, and what alternative exists if the family can no longer continue.

Hospital - Security and Technology Alongside the Risk of Therapeutic Inertia

A hospital is not necessarily an undignified place to die. For some people it provides a sense of safety, immediate access to staff, the ability to control difficult symptoms, and relief for relatives who cannot carry the responsibility at home. In a palliative unit or a ward that understands the goals of care, a person can die quietly in hospital with family present, symptoms controlled, and unwanted interventions avoided.

The hospital risk is inertia. A change in vital signs can automatically trigger a chain of tests, infusions, and transfers because the system is built for action. If the goal of care is not documented and communicated across shifts, a person who asked for comfort-focused care can be pulled back into an aggressive pathway. Quality end-of-life care in hospital therefore depends less on the ward's name than on making the goal visible: what continues, what does not, who speaks with the family, and what happens when the condition deteriorates.

Inpatient Hospice and Long-Term Care - Options Between Home and Hospital

Inpatient hospice combines palliative expertise with an environment that is not oriented toward acute intervention at all costs. For a person without sufficient support at home or with complex symptoms, it may be the best option. Its limitations are availability, distance from family, and number of beds. A declared right to choose has little meaning if no hospice bed is actually available in the region where the person lives.

Long-term care institutions are the homes of many people for months or years, so transfer to hospital near the end of life is not always the best default. A team that knows the person may sometimes provide comfort in the familiar setting if resources, medication, and clear instructions are available. At the same time, age or place of residence must never become a reason to withhold reversible treatment the person wants and that can benefit them. Place should operate together with treatment goals, not replace clinical judgment.

Preference for Place Is a Dynamic Decision

Research on place of death shows that preferences are influenced by illness, support, available services, and prior experience. Someone who has never seen a hospice may imagine home as the only place of safety and later change his or her mind after experiencing hospice care. Another person may want to remain at home while still able to communicate and choose hospital when a frightening symptom develops. The question of place should therefore be revisited rather than answered once and frozen for months.

How the question is asked also matters. "Where would you like to die?" is a heavy question and may come too early. It may be better to begin with, "Where would you want to be if your condition worsened?" or "What would need to be in place for you to remain at home?" This turns preference into a plan rather than a symbol. The conversation should also permit the answer that the person has no strong preference; that too is legitimate.

Equality - Who Can Truly Choose?

Choosing home depends on resources. An accessible apartment, a relative able to remain present, the ability to absorb lost workdays, proximity to services, and the ability to navigate the health system all affect whether a preference can be realized. If only people with available family and resources can die at home, a policy celebrating higher rates of home death may conceal inequality. The state should provide home services and respite so that preference does not become a privilege.

The primary caregiver also has limits. Patient autonomy does not compel a partner to perform care that the partner is unable to sustain. A conversation about place of death should explore what the patient wants and what the surrounding support network can realistically provide, then construct an alternative that respects both as far as possible. Sometimes hospice or hospital is the more dignified option precisely because it allows a relative to return to being a spouse or child rather than remain only an exhausted caregiver.

What, Then, Is "Death with Dignity"?

The phrase "death with dignity" is used by opposing camps to support contrary conclusions. For one, it means control over the time and manner of death; for another, it means recognition that human life retains value even in complete dependence. The phrase alone therefore cannot decide the issue. Yet practical conditions can be identified on which most perspectives should be able to agree: do not leave a person in treatable pain; do not conceal information the person asks to receive; do not impose treatment the person rejects when the law recognizes the right to refuse; do not abandon a person who has chosen not to prolong life; and do not turn the body into a space in which the system acts without regard to the person's values.

Dignity can include the possibility of being at home, but dignity is not synonymous with home. It includes privacy, relief, communication, presence, humane treatment, and the ability to choose what can still be chosen. A person can die at home and feel abandoned if pain is uncontrolled; another can die in hospital and feel respected if the team knows the person, explains what is happening, protects the body, and allows loved ones to be present. Place shapes the experience, but the way the system behaves within that place determines its quality.

In this sense, the book's final clinical question is not where it is right to die, nor which technology is right. It is whether the health system can change its purpose when reality changes: from the effort to cure to the effort to relieve; from control of disease to preservation of the person. End of life is not the moment when medicine stops. It is the moment when medicine is tested on whether it knows how to continue caring even when it can no longer promise rescue.

The Ambulance and the Emergency Department - Where a Plan Can Break

Even an excellent home plan is tested in a crisis. A family member sees altered breathing or decreased consciousness and calls emergency services. The ambulance crew meets a person it does not know, under time pressure, often without immediate access to all relevant documents. If the goals of care are not clear and accessible, the natural default is intervention and transport to hospital. Within minutes, a pathway the patient hoped to avoid may begin.

Planning the place of death should therefore include an emergency plan: who calls the hospice team, which symptoms are expected, what can be given at home, when transfer is desired, and which document can be recognized quickly by an outside team. The goal is not to prevent transport at any cost; in some situations hospital is the correct choice. The goal is for transfer to result from need and preference rather than from lack of information.

The emergency department can also be a point of correction. Before escalating to aggressive treatment, where circumstances permit, staff can pause to determine whether directives exist, who knows the patient's wishes, and what the goal of care was in the community. Minutes for clarification are not always available during active resuscitation, but in many cases there is a window in which inertia can be prevented. Digital infrastructure that surfaces a short, reliable document may be more valuable than another form stored at home.

The Moment of Death and What Happens Immediately Afterward

Quality care does not end at the moment death is declared. How the team informs relatives, allows them to remain with the body, respects religious and cultural practices, and explains what will happen next can shape the family's memory of the event. Even an expected death can be overwhelming. Quiet, privacy, and avoidance of unnecessary activity are part of the respect the system shows both the person and those close to them.

At home, the family needs clear instructions about whom to contact after death and what to expect. In hospital, it needs time that is not dictated solely by the pressure to free a bed. When organ donation may be possible or a legal investigation is required, the process can be more complex, but it can still be explained in humane language. The final test of end-of-life care is not only how the medical decision was made, but how the system remained present after medical treatment itself had ended.

The Gap Between the Preferred Place and the Place Where Death Occurs

Research on place of death examines not only what people say they want but also the match between preference and the place where they actually die. A mismatch may result from changing wishes, clinical deterioration, loss of a home caregiver, service availability, or an emergency event. A mismatch is therefore not always a failure; the important question is whether the plan changed by choice or broke because of a system limitation.

A sound quality measure should distinguish between the two. If a person changed his or her mind and requested hospitalization, death in hospital may be consistent with the most recent wish. If the person wanted to remain at home but no night service or appropriate equipment was available, the same outcome tells a story about access. The variable "place of death" alone is insufficient; it should be linked to a preference documented as close as possible to the event and to the reason the plan changed.

This distinction matters for policy because a high rate of home death may look positive even when families carry an unreasonable burden, while a high rate of hospital death may look negative even when some patients chose it. Quality is not a geographic target but a match among wishes, need, and infrastructure.

Geography, Housing, and the Periphery - When the Preferred Place Is Not Equally Accessible

The ability to choose a place of care and death also depends on the physical environment. A small apartment without an elevator, a home into which a bed or equipment cannot be brought, a long distance from a palliative team, or lack of transport can make a principled preference for home impractical. Sometimes the question is not whether the patient wants to remain at home, but whether the home can become a safe place of care without destroying privacy or placing an intolerable burden on the family.

The gap is especially visible between central and peripheral regions and between areas in which home care is rapidly available and those in which a team must travel a long distance. When there is no after-hours response, an event that a stronger system might manage at home can lead to transfer. Palliative-service planning therefore must include not only staffing numbers but response time, night coverage, access to medication, and remote consultation. Telemedicine does not replace a visit when touch, examination, or treatment is required, but it can prevent an unnecessary transfer when the family needs immediate guidance.

A residence that is not a private home also requires individualized thinking. A person living alone, in assisted living, in a nursing home, or with relatives may define "home" differently from an administrative definition. Policy should look at where the person actually lives and who can support them rather than assume one concept of home fits everyone. For someone who has lived for years in a long-term care institution, transfer to hospital may itself mean removal from the familiar place; for another, that institution may be unable to provide the needed care.

Equality in this field therefore requires more than a formal right to choose. It requires the system to ask what conditions are missing for the choice to become possible. Sometimes the answer is equipment, sometimes nursing hours, sometimes medication, and sometimes another option such as inpatient hospice. A policy that records only the preference but not why it could not be realized misses the point at which services can actually be improved.

Support Does Not End When Death Is Declared

In a system that provides good end-of-life care, the family does not instantly move from being the companion of a patient to being outside the system. Brief information about the next steps, a chance to ask questions, direction to bereavement services when appropriate, and follow-up in complex situations can prevent a sense of abrupt abandonment after a period in which the team was intensely present.

Bereavement support does not require turning every death into prolonged therapy. Most people will move through grief with family and community support. The system's role is to identify situations in which the risk of significant difficulty is higher: traumatic death, severe conflict over treatment, a child who has lost a parent, an isolated partner, or intense guilt. In such circumstances, proactive referral can be part of responsible continuity of care.

The team may also need closure. A prolonged case, a strong relationship with a family, or a moral conflict can leave a mark. A brief team discussion after a difficult event allows learning without blame: what worked, what failed to pass between shifts, whether the patient's wishes were clear, and what might be done differently next time. In that way, the death of one patient can become a source of improvement in care for the next.

Cultural and religious practices after death may also deserve advance planning when they matter to the person. Different families may ask for prayer, presence of clergy, particular treatment of the body, rapid burial, or time for farewell before transfer. A hospital cannot guarantee every request, especially when legal or medical limits apply, but it can ask what matters, explain what is possible, and reduce conflicts that otherwise arise at the most sensitive moment. Cultural adaptation here is not abandonment of rules; it is a way of applying them without erasing the person's identity when the person can no longer speak for himself or herself.

Conclusion

Between the Ability to Prolong Life and the Duty to Know When to Let Go

Modern medicine has given humanity a power unavailable to most earlier generations: an ever-growing ability to influence the boundary between life and death. That power has saved millions of lives, but it has also transformed the final stage of life into a field of decisions that did not previously exist. When it is possible to ventilate, resuscitate, dialyze, provide artificial nutrition, and continue treatment for long periods, technical possibility alone does not answer whether an intervention serves the person.

The journey in this book began long before Israeli law. It moved through ancient understandings of suffering and death, the development of medical ethics, the rise of autonomy, and the technological revolution that turned the end of life into a domain of choice. From there, the discussion moved to the concepts that allow precise analysis: capacity, prognosis, life-prolonging treatment, life-saving treatment, palliative care, sedation, withholding treatment, withdrawing treatment, assisted dying, and euthanasia. These distinctions are not an academic exercise; they are the condition for giving a clinical decision the correct legal meaning.

Law can establish a framework, but it cannot replace professional judgment. Determining that a person meets the legal definition of a dying patient rests on medical assessment. Evaluating capacity requires attention to reversible factors such as delirium, pain, medications, or metabolic disturbance. Interpreting an earlier wish requires understanding the context in which it was expressed. And a decision not to begin a particular treatment does not abolish the duty to continue caring for the person. When the process is done well, law and clinical medicine reinforce each other. When it is done superficially, even a clear statutory provision can fail at the bedside.

At precisely this point, the importance of nursing becomes visible. The nurse is not merely the executor of a decision made elsewhere. Often, the nurse stands at the point where a decision becomes an act: observing breathing, pain, agitation, family reaction, functional change, and the gap between a general order and a new situation. Accurate nursing documentation, handoff between shifts, and timely escalation of doubt are part of the mechanism protecting the patient. In a future legal dispute, that record may also reconstruct reality in a way that no later memory can.

Law cannot eliminate the tragedy of the end of life. It can prevent coercion, allocate authority, create mechanisms for resolving disputes, and mark boundaries. It cannot guarantee the absence of pain, guilt, or disagreement among relatives. The best law is therefore not one that promises an easy answer in every case, but one that requires a fair, transparent, professional process and protects both the individual's wishes and those who may be vulnerable to pressure, error, or neglect.

International comparison has shown that no single model provides an answer for every society. The Netherlands, Belgium, Canada, U.S. states, Australia, New Zealand, and South American jurisdictions have built different frameworks, while other countries have chosen primarily to expand recognition of refusal of treatment and advance directives. Even where there is agreement on values such as dignity, compassion, and autonomy, there need not be agreement on the legal conclusion. The difference often lies in which danger the state seeks more strongly to prevent: life being imposed against a person's wishes, or life being lost through a process that is insufficiently protected.

There is therefore little value in ending the discussion by declaring that autonomy has defeated sanctity of life, or vice versa. A humane society must hold both values at the same time. Autonomy without protection can leave a vulnerable person exposed to pressure; protection of life without listening to the person's wishes can become paternalism that prolongs suffering against the patient's position. The true test of the system is its ability to identify the individual case rather than hide behind a slogan.

In Israel, the Dying Patient Law is a distinctive attempt to construct this balance. It is not the end of the discussion. Changes in medicine, technology, demography, and law require periodic examination of whether the mechanisms remain accessible and whether the distinctions built into the law still achieve their purposes. Even if the prohibition on active euthanasia remains unchanged, there is substantial room for improvement: earlier conversations, more accessible directives, palliative care, professional training, high-quality documentation, coordination between community and hospital care, and rapid mechanisms for resolving disputes.

For readers approaching the field from a legal perspective, perhaps the most important lesson is that medical responsibility at the end of life does not begin in the courtroom. It begins much earlier: in an explanation given on time, a question asked, a doubt documented, reassessment of capacity, a distinction between reversible treatment and treatment that no longer achieves its goal, and the team's knowledge of what the person asked for before losing the ability to speak. When the system functions in this way, law is not merely an instrument of retrospective criticism; it becomes part of good treatment planning.

For readers approaching the field from medicine or nursing, law offers a parallel reminder: good intentions alone are not enough. Professional power requires boundaries, consent, documentation, and the ability to explain why a particular course was chosen. Precisely when clinicians are convinced that they are acting in a patient's best interests, they must ask whether that conception of benefit also reflects the person's values and wishes, rather than only the professionals' own view.

In the end, not every death can be made "good." Some illnesses are devastating, some farewells come too early, and some suffering has no complete solution. But a system can still strive not to add avoidable suffering; not to let the person disappear behind machines; not to leave a family alone with a decision it does not understand; and not to force professionals to choose between compassion and law because the system failed to give them a language and practical tools.

This may be the deepest challenge of end-of-life medicine: to distinguish between giving up on the person and giving up an intervention that no longer serves that person. Death is not medicine's failure. Abandoning the person in the face of death is the failure to be avoided.

Short Glossary of Terms

The glossary is intended for orientation only. Full definitions, qualifications, and differences between Israeli law and other legal systems are discussed in the relevant chapters.

Dying patient - A specific legal category under Israeli law; it should not be used as a synonym for every seriously ill person or every person with an incurable disease.

Capacity - The ability to understand relevant information, appreciate its significance in relation to one's own situation, weigh alternatives, and communicate a choice. Capacity is assessed in relation to the particular decision.

Advance medical directives - Instructions given by a person while competent in order to express wishes for the future if the person later cannot make or communicate a decision.

Power of attorney - A mechanism through which a person appoints someone in advance to express the person's wishes and act within the authority granted by law if capacity is lost.

Life-saving treatment - An intervention intended to address a life-threatening condition when there is a realistic possibility of changing the course and achieving clinical benefit.

Life-prolonging treatment - An intervention that may prolong life or the dying process; its meaning depends on its purpose, context, expected benefit, and burden for the particular patient.

Palliative care - Active care intended to reduce suffering and improve quality of life through symptom treatment, communication, and support for the patient and family.

Withholding treatment - A decision not to begin a particular medical intervention. It does not mean stopping all care or abandoning the patient.

Withdrawing treatment - Ending an intervention that has already begun. Its legal and ethical significance varies according to the type and purpose of treatment and the applicable law.

Continuous and cyclical treatment - A central distinction in Israeli law between treatment that operates continuously and treatment delivered in doses or cycles requiring renewal.

Palliative sedation - Reduction of consciousness in order to relieve severe refractory symptoms within palliative care, with the purpose of relieving suffering rather than causing death.

Active euthanasia - An intentional act in which a professional causes a person's death at that person's request within a legal system that permits the practice; it is not permitted in Israel.

Medical assistance in dying - A broad term whose meaning varies among jurisdictions; it may include a pathway in which a professional provides the means and the individual performs the final act.

Do-not-resuscitate order (DNR) - An order not to perform resuscitation in the event of cardiac or respiratory arrest. It is not an instruction to stop other treatment and is not equivalent to "do not treat."

Foundational Sources and Framework for Academic Updating

This list brings together the principal primary, institutional, and research sources on which the book relies. Footnotes have been incorporated at central points of argument in the body of the book. In the print edition, citation style should remain consistent with the publisher's requirements, and legislation, case law, and changing regulatory arrangements should be checked for currency close to publication.

1. Israel - Dying Patient Law, 5766-2005, together with the regulations and forms issued under it.

2. Israel - Patients' Rights Law, 5756-1996.

3. Israel Ministry of Health - Advance Medical Directives and Power of Attorney service, the national database, and updated public information (updated May 2026).

4. Israel Ministry of Health - Public Committee on the Dying Patient (the Steinberg Committee), reports and recommendations.

5. Knesset Research and Information Center - documents concerning implementation of the Dying Patient Law, palliative care, and advance medical directives, including the March 2025 report.

6. World Health Organization - policy sources and guidance concerning palliative care.

7. World Medical Association - declarations concerning euthanasia, physician-assisted suicide, and medical care at the end of life.

8. Netherlands - Termination of Life on Request and Assisted Suicide (Review Procedures) Act; government sources and Regional Euthanasia Review Committees reports, including the 2025 report published in March 2026.

9. Belgium - Act on Euthanasia; Federal Commission for the Control and Evaluation of Euthanasia, including 2025 data published in March 2026.

10. Luxembourg - Law of 16 March 2009 on euthanasia and assisted suicide, and official health-system guidance.

11. Spain - Organic Law 3/2021 of 24 March 2021 regulating euthanasia, and official implementation documents.

12. Switzerland - provisions of the Criminal Code and official and legal sources concerning assistance in suicide.

13. Germany - Federal Constitutional Court, judgment of 26 February 2020 concerning the right to a self-determined death.

14. Italy - Constitutional Court case law and legislative sources concerning assisted suicide and refusal of treatment.

15. France - Law No. 2026-404 of 26 May 2026 concerning accompaniment and palliative care; National Assembly and Constitutional Council materials concerning the assisted-dying proposal referred for constitutional review in July 2026.

16. United Kingdom - Parliament and House of Commons Library, Terminally Ill Adults (End of Life) Bills; the 2024-2026 proposal that failed and the 2026-2027 proposal whose second reading was scheduled for 11 September 2026.

17. Canada - Criminal Code, Department of Justice, and Health Canada materials concerning MAID; note the exclusion of mental illness as the sole underlying medical condition until 17 March 2027.

18. United States - state legislation and official sources concerning medical aid in dying, including the entry into force of New York State's Medical Aid in Dying law on 5 August 2026, together with the principal federal constitutional case law.

19. Colombia - Constitutional Court and Ministry of Health sources concerning the right to die with dignity and euthanasia, including Resolución 813 de 2026.

20. Ecuador - Constitutional Court, Judgment 67-23-IN/24, and later official sources.

21. Uruguay - Law No. 20.431, enacted 24 October 2025 and published 5 November 2025; Decree 76/026 of 15 April 2026 and the government protocol adopted under them.

22. Argentina - Law 26.742 and official sources concerning patient autonomy, refusal of treatment, and advance directives.

23. Australia - voluntary assisted dying laws in the states and territories, regulations, and health-authority guidance; in Victoria, amendments approved in November 2025 are scheduled to take effect in April 2027.

24. New Zealand - End of Life Choice Act 2019; Ministry of Health regulatory materials and the Registrar's annual report published in July 2026 covering the period through 31 March 2026.

25. India - Supreme Court, Cause Common and subsequent case law, including Harish Rana v. Union of India, 2026 INSC 222 (11 March 2026), concerning withholding and withdrawal of life-prolonging treatment and advance directives.

26. Singapore - Advance Medical Directive Act and Ministry of Health guidance.

27. Taiwan - Patient Right to Autonomy Act and official legislative-database sources.

28. South Korea - Act on Decisions on Life-Sustaining Treatment for Patients in Hospice and Palliative Care or at the End of Life.

29. South Africa - Supreme Court of Appeal decision in Stransham-Ford (2016) and Law Reform Commission materials.

30. European Court of Human Rights - relevant case law concerning private life, refusal of treatment, and assisted dying.

31. Council of Europe - Convention on Human Rights and Biomedicine and related bioethics sources.

32. Austria - Sterbeverfügungsgesetz-Novelle 2026; Austrian parliamentary proceedings in July 2026, including the renewal provision scheduled to take effect on 1 February 2027.

Selected Research Literature for Further Academic Study

Beauchamp TL, Childress JF. Principles of Biomedical Ethics. 8th ed. Oxford University Press; 2019.

Steinberg A, Sprung CL. The Dying Patient Act, 2005: Israeli Innovative Legislation. Israel Medical Association Journal. 2007;9:550-552.

Emanuel EJ, Onwuteaka-Philipsen BD, Urwin JW, Cohen J. Attitudes and Practices of Euthanasia and Physician-Assisted Suicide in the United States, Canada, and Europe. JAMA. 2016;316(1):79-90.

Battin MP, van der Heide A, Ganzini L, van der Wal G, Onwuteaka-Philipsen BD. Legal physician-assisted dying in Oregon and the Netherlands: evidence concerning the impact on patients in vulnerable groups. Journal of Medical Ethics. 2007;33(10):591-597.

Grove G, Lovell M, Best M. Perspectives of Major World Religions regarding Euthanasia and Assisted Suicide: A Comparative Analysis. Journal of Religion and Health. 2022;61:4758-4782.

McCormick AJ. Buddhist Ethics and End-of-Life Care Decisions. Journal of Social Work in End-of-Life & Palliative Care. 2013;9(2-3):209-225.

Sharma H et al. End-of-life care: Indian perspective. Indian Journal of Psychiatry. 2013;55(Suppl 2):S293-S298.

Yang Y et al. Confucian Familism and Shared Decision Making in End-of-Life Care for Patients with Advanced Cancers. International Journal of Environmental Research and Public Health. 2022;19.

World Health Organization. Palliative care; guidance on access to controlled medicines and morphine. Current online sources accessed for this edition.

Cherny NI, Radbruch L. European Association for Palliative Care (EAPC) recommended framework for the use of sedation in palliative care. Palliative Medicine. 2009;23(7):581-593.

Surges SM et al. Revised European Association for Palliative Care (EAPC) recommended framework on palliative sedation: an international Delphi study. Palliative Medicine. 2024.

Appelbaum PS, Grisso T. Assessing patients' capacities to consent to treatment. New England Journal of Medicine. 1988;319:1635-1638.

Grisso T, Appelbaum PS, Hill-Fotouhi C. The MacCAT-T: a clinical tool to assess patients' capacities to make treatment decisions. Psychiatric Services. 1997;48(11):1415-1419.

Block SD, Billings JA. Patient requests to hasten death: evaluation and management in terminal care. Archives of Internal Medicine. 1994;154(18):2039-2047.

Breitbart W et al. Depression, hopelessness, and desire for hastened death in terminally ill patients with cancer. JAMA. 2000;284:2907-2911.

Balaguer A et al. An international consensus definition of the wish to hasten death and its related factors. PLoS ONE. 2016.

Bernacki RE, Block SD. Communication about serious illness care goals: a review and synthesis of best practices. JAMA Internal Medicine. 2014;174(12):1994-2003.

Rachels J. Active and passive euthanasia. New England Journal of Medicine. 1975;292:78-80.

Zigdon A et al. Barriers in implementing the Dying Patient Law: the Israeli experience. BMC Medical Ethics. 2020.

Bentur N et al. The attitudes of physicians toward the new Dying Patient Act enacted in Israel. American Journal of Hospice & Palliative Medicine. 2008.

Additional Sources for the Expanded Edition

Israel Ministry of Health, Committee for Determination of Brain-Respiratory Death and the Brain-Respiratory Death Determination Law, 5768-2008; updated information and guidance on the Ministry of Health website.

American Academy of Neurology. Practice Guideline Update Recommendations: Disorders of Consciousness. 2018; reaffirmed 2024.

World Medical Association. Declaration of Venice on End of Life Medical Care. Revised 2022.

World Medical Association. Declaration on Euthanasia and Physician-Assisted Suicide. 2019.

American Medical Association Code of Medical Ethics, Opinion 5.3: Withholding or Withdrawing Life-Sustaining Treatment.

Knesset Research and Information Center. Implementation of the Dying Patient Law. 9 March 2025.

Israel Ministry of Health. Advance Medical Directives and Power of Attorney; Care of the Dying Patient; Palliative Care. Public information, 2026.

Pinto S, et al. Patient and Family Preferences About Place of End-of-Life Care and Death: An Umbrella Review. Journal of Pain and Symptom Management. 2024;67(5):e439-e452.

Farinha-Costa B, Reis-Pina P. Home Hospitalization in Palliative Care for Advanced Cancer and Dementia: A Systematic Review. Journal of Pain and Symptom Management. 2025;69(3):289-303.

Giachello M et al. Communication Tools for End-of-Life Conversations in Palliative Nursing. American Journal of Hospice & Palliative Care. 2026;43(8):892-899.

Gomes B et al. Preferences for place of death if faced with advanced cancer: a population survey in England, Flanders, Germany, Italy, the Netherlands, Portugal and Spain. Annals of Oncology. 2012;23:2006-2015.

Gomes B et al. Heterogeneity and changes in preferences for dying at home: a systematic review. BMC Palliative Care. 2013.

www.ingramcontent.com/pod-product-compliance
Lightning Source LLC
LaVergne TN
LVHW010714061126
851857LV00014B/1182
9789659339723